PATIENT SATISFACTION in SPINE PRACTICE

Review of Literatures and Personal Experience

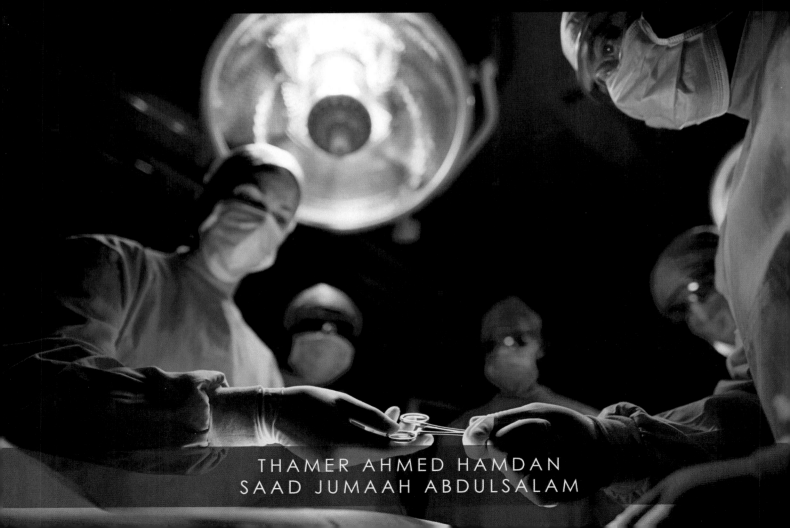

THAMER AHMED HAMDAN
SAAD JUMAAH ABDULSALAM

AuthorHouse™ UK
1663 Liberty Drive
Bloomington, IN 47403 USA
www.authorhouse.co.uk
UK TFN: 0800 0148641 (Toll Free inside the UK)
UK Local: 02036 956322 (+44 20 3695 6322 from outside the UK)

Because of the dynamic nature of the Internet, any web addresses or links contained in this book may have changed since publication and may no longer be valid. The views expressed in this work are solely those of the author and do not necessarily reflect the views of the publisher, and the publisher hereby disclaims any responsibility for them.

Any people depicted in stock imagery provided by Getty Images are models, and such images are being used for illustrative purposes only.
Certain stock imagery © Getty Images.

This book is printed on acid-free paper.

ISBN: 978-1-7283-5435-4 (sc)
ISBN: 978-1-7283-5434-7 (e)

Print information available on the last page.

Published by AuthorHouse 09/23/2020

authorHOUSE®

Dedication

This book is dedicated to our dear patients with complex spinal pathology.

To our dear colleagues;

The spinal surgeons all over the Globe, particularly those working with poor theater facilities...

And to Lord and Lady Swinfen for their outstanding work to satisfy patients all over the Globe, without restriction...

Preface

Hopefully all colleagues in spinal practice, realize, how difficult to achieve perfection in spinal practice, this is related to the varieties of treatment, the complexities of the spinal pathology, and the difference in opinion about even one pathology.

Probably as important as the treatment is achieving patient satisfaction, I think almost all spinal surgeons are happy with this conclusion.

So the motive behind writing this book is to keep our dear colleagues fully aware of this vital issue, we have to work hard to achieve satisfaction even before cure.

From my practice I have seen some patients fully satisfied though they did not achieve cure, and the reverse is true.

So many articles were written about patient satisfaction but so far no book was written in the English literatures.

Hopefully this book will be a guideline to proper handling of our dear patients in regard to achieving satisfaction as much as possible.

T. A. Hamdan

Contents

Dedication. iii

Preface v

Introduction. xi

I.   PATIENT SATISFACTION PRINCIPLES 1

   Patient Satisfaction. 1

   Key concepts of patient experience 1

   Patient experience and patient safety 2

   Patient Satisfaction and the Quality of Care 2

   Care and Service 3

   Care or Cure? 6

   The Link to Quality 7

   Quality assessment. 7

   Trust Enhancement 8

   Importance of Communication. 8

   Stress Reduction 9

   The Placebo Effect 9

   Safety and Satisfaction 10

   Action for Satisfaction. 11

   The link to Employee Satisfaction. 11

   The link to Physician Satisfaction. 12

   Patient expectations 14

II. AIDET 15

AIDET and professionalism..15

The importance of keywords 16

A: Acknowledge; Safety and respect...............................17

I: Introduce; Decrease anxiety, building trust to increase compliance 17

D: Duration;..18

E: Explanation.... Quality 18

T: Thank You, Patient loyalty 19

Post Discharge Phone Calls 19

Nurse Hourly Rounding 20

Leader Rounding..20

III. PATIENT REPORTED OUTCOME 22

Patient reported satisfaction and its impact on outcomes in spinal surgery 25

Involving patients in system design 27

Patient experience of care 27

Waiting time..29

Successful Strategies for Waiting Rooms 29

Pain management...30

Family involvement 31

Empathy...32

Patient's listening 33

Hospital length of stay...33

IV. THE HCAHPS...34

HCAHPS Fact Sheet 34

Overview 34

HCAHPS Development, Testing and Endorsement............35

HCAHPS Survey Content and Administration..................35

HCAHPS Measures...36

What do patients want from the healthcare provider? 37

Common Challenges 38

Improving Response Rate Strategies 38

Overall HCAHPS Success strategies 38

Communication with Nurses 39

Key Strategies 39

Communication with Physicians 39

Responsiveness of hospital staff 40

Hourly Rounding 41

No Pass Zone 41

Technological Devices 41

Pain Management 41

Communication about Medications 42

Cleanliness of Hospital Environment 43

Quietness of Hospital Environment 44

Discharge Information 44

Discharge Planning 45

Discharge Phone Calls or Home Visits 45

Care Transitions Strategies 45

Patient-centered care organizational status checklist 46

What must hospitals do in order to participate in HCAHPS? 47

Which patients are eligible to participate in HCAHPS? 47

V. SATISFACTION AND PATIENTS WITH SPINE DISEASES 49

Patient Selection for Spine Surgery 49

Patient expectations 50

Microendoscopic Diskectomy 52

Smoking 53

Preoperative diagnosis 54

Obesity 55

Coronary artery disease 56

Gender. 57

Psychological status. 57

ASA class 57

Fusion surgery 58

Scoliosis 59

Patient age 60

Open and MIS. 63

Motion preserving surgery. 64

Spinal stenosis 67

References. 71

Appendix I. 85

Introduction

To treat or to satisfy the patient; which one is the best?

Luckily, there is increasing interest in patient satisfaction in the present days. Many writers started differentiating between the two issues; treatment or satisfaction. Patient satisfaction is a top priority and it should be the target. Perfect treatment is not always satisfactory to the patient. Some surgeons, sadly, spoil their ideal treatment by misconduct. They are good enough to offer treatment, but not good enough in performing the art of communication, which is really vital. They do not know how to respect the dignity, the honor and rights of the patient. The first meeting is the key for success in achieving life-long friendship or, on the other hand "putting salt on the wound"

The art of patient handling is not that easy. Surgeon's words, sometimes, create emergency, probably much more serious than the surgeon's knife. What looks minor to the Surgeon may be enough to make the patient complaining bitterly.

Several points and steps are, therefore, required to achieve appropriate satisfaction. As cited above, performing highly skilled and perfect surgery is not enough to satisfy the patient, since satisfaction is a complex issue that depends on several parameters. Sound judgment, high index of patient selection, surgeon's behavior, sympathy and empathy, feeling patient's suffering, and surgeon's skills are all required.

The surgeon's behavior is the key for success or failure. He is the first to be blamed even for problems not related to him, because, in the patient's mind, he is considered to be the leader.

In addition, the administrative and paper works, patient's transportation, the buildings and sanitary facilities, and the ward environment; how clean and fresh it is, all are basic requirements for satisfaction in the mind of patients and their escorts. Moreover, the nursing staff; how they handle the patient and how they follow the patient status, are also another factor contributing to patient's satisfaction. They should be very sympathetic in all aspects.

Listening to patient's suffering is very vital, and is required from all partners in the treatment team. Some pathological processes require prolonged treatment and may be associated with prolonged suffering. So, proper handling and utmost care is mandatory. We have to treat the patient psyche before treating the physical illness. No way of showing or using any pattern of force. It is very irritating even if ideal treatment is offered. Smooth, quiet and comforting words are mandatory.

The structure and design of the accommodation, also, have an impact on the patient's mind. Some patients need very special handling, like those who are already psychologically traumatized, those with incurable conditions, prolonged illnesses, recurrent pathologies, previous mishandling or those who are badly treated by other colleagues. All the above may be troublesome and very difficult to satisfy. Patients' escorts are, sometimes, worse than patients themselves.

Alleviating pain, by any mean, will induce confidence and satisfaction; also relieving other symptoms like fever, diarrhea, or vomiting. Prolonged waiting list will induce fed up, and necessitates cares on behalf of the surgeon and the hospital.

Age and gender may make some difference in the patients' satisfaction. In my experience, the teenager girls are not easy to satisfy.

In our locality, there is a break in the doctor-patient relationship which contributes, to a great extent, for not achieving satisfaction. We have to work hard to improve our behavior towards our dear patients. Our handling of patients' needs revision. Courses are required to teach young generations how to behave to achieve satisfaction. A questionnaire is required to spot the weak points in handling patients before leaving the hospital. This will help very much. Follow up is part of the patient's treatment. It has a real impact on patient's satisfaction.

Finally, it is never enough to offer treatment alone. Satisfaction should go hand-in-hand with the ideal treatment.

I

Patient Satisfaction Principles

Patient Satisfaction

Satisfaction; A pleasant feeling that you get when you receive something you wanted, or when you have done something you wanted to do. Or ... A way of dealing with a complaint or problem that makes the person who complained feel happy. A situation in which your complaint or problem is dealt with in a way you consider acceptable. If something is done to someone's satisfaction, they are happy with the result [1].

It also can be defined as culmination or meeting of expectations of a person from a service or product. When a patient comes to a hospital, he has a predetermined image of the various aspects of the hospital as per the reputation and cost involved. Although, their main expectation is getting cured and going back to their work, but there are other elements, which affect their satisfaction [2].

Key concepts of patient experience

- ❖ Patient experience goes exceeding satisfaction and "making patients happy."
- ❖ You may have a negative result but still have a positive patient experience.
- ❖ You may have a positive result but a negative patient experience.
- ❖ Patient experience is linked employee engagement
- ❖ Patients judge healthcare providers not only on clinical outcomes, but also sympathize and excellent, patient centered care [3,4].

Patient experience and patient safety

When physicians communicate better, synchronization of care improves and compliance with treatment modes increases. Those are quality issues. When nurses communicate effectively at the bedside, medication errors go down, pressure ulcers go down, and falls go down. Those are safety issues.

A small but increasing body of evidence shows the link between aspects of patient experience and clinical quality. Anxiety and fear delay healing but are relieved by emotional and psychological support [3,4].

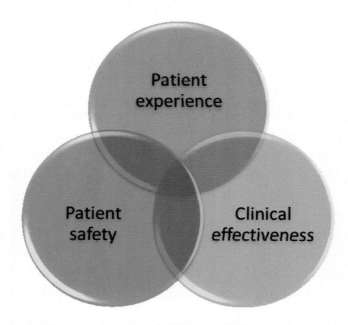

Patient Satisfaction and the Quality of Care

Human satisfaction is a very complex notion that is stirred by a number of factors like lifestyle, past experience, future expectation and the belief of individual and society in terms of ethical and economical standings.

Knowledge of expectation and the factors affecting them, combined with knowledge of real and perceived healthcare quality, provides the vital information for designing and fulfilling programs to satisfy patients [2].

Patient satisfaction can be an integral strategy for achieving and sustaining the mission of the institution.

When patient satisfaction taken very seriously, there will be;

> ➤ Higher quality of care;
> ➤ Staff will be more gratified with their jobs, and turnover will be lower;
> ➤ The institution will be more likely to stay financially strong
> ➤ The competitive position will be powerful
> ➤ Workers in health services less likely to be litigated [4,5].

Care and Service

Hospitals have evolved from being an isolated infirmary to a place with five star facilities. The patients and their relatives coming to the hospital not only expect world-class treatment, but also other facilities to make their stay comfortable in the hospital.

Many healthcare professionals still feel that patients may be able to assess service but not technical-medical care. If the food is bad, then they might rate the whole spectrum of care lower.

Service and care are distinct entities, they might combat. Do not be confused with the two.

Care; Is a direct technical intervention (emphasis on "technical"), this is the key.

Service. Is a peripheral, interpersonal and existential. To such professionals, "service" suggests that treating customers rather than patients. This affects their professional identity.

Service is often viewed as a matter of personality and pleasantness.

Such views have led to simplistic approaches to dealing with patient satisfaction.

Direct measures ask about the patient's personal experiences with health care, and indirect measures ask about the patient's attitudes toward health care and the health care system in general [4,5].

Most service-focused programs have not changed much from the guest-relations efforts of the 1980s, which staff often labeled as "smile school."

> ➤ Look to the patient in the eye when talking.
> ➤ Introduce yourself.
> ➤ Sit next to the patient rather than stand at the foot of the bed.
> ➤ Be respectful, be caring (whatever that means) and prompt.
> ➤ Reduce delays.
> ➤ Keep the soup hot and the carpets clean.

Care, on the other hand, is often viewed as having to do with IV lines, medication, treatment explanations, postoperative instructions, and other technical or informational interventions.

In fact, the service/care distinction is an attention drawing issue.

It's all service, and it's all care. The form in which care is provided defines, for the patient, the nature and effectiveness of that care.

Amenity, attitudes, information, explanations, body language, physical touch, tidy sounds and sights— all these factors have an effect on the patient's experience of care.

If patients perceive the carpets to be soiled, or corridor noise excessive, or the nurses less than friendly, then will it impact their experience of care? Notice I said "experience" of care, not care itself.

The difference is significant. From the patient's side, care involves everything that goes on, everything that is experienced.

Every view, sound, interaction, and intervention impact to the overall experience and is interpreted as a purposeful side of care. No patient wants to think that anything unplanned happens in the vicinity of his care.

The patient is in a strange place with strange and anxiety producing rituals. Stress and disorientation is common.

If the nurse fails to provide adequate reassurance or information as she attempts to insert the IV, is this an issue of service or care?

If her appearance, body language, or manner do not communicate empathy as she sticks the patient, is this a care or service issue? What about food? For many patients, the simple, familiar, nurturing ritual of meal time provides some feeling of groundedness. If the meal is delayed or if it is unattractively prepared, is this a failure of service or care? Again, to the patient, there is no way to distinguish between the two. Everything the hospital or clinic does is defined as care.

What do patients want from healthcare; technical quality or service quality?

We all want the highest quality of technical (clinical) care. Technical care is a necessary criterion for judging care overall. At the same time, it is only a partial—and thus insufficient—criterion for making this judgment [4,6,7].

Patients do judge the quality of clinical care they receive. However, they base their judgments on far more than the technical interventions, many of which they are unaware. Patients cannot judge whether the proper gauge needle is being used for the injection, whether 10 cc is the proper dose, or whether heparin is the proper medication. But patients can judge whether the injection hurt more than anticipated, whether the nurse was informative as well as friendly, or whether the doctor listened to the patient's ideas and questions and responded appropriately.

Moreover, if patients sense that physicians are not interested in them or are not concerned with good communication or empathy, then they doubt the physicians' ability to actually use their full competence. Patients would then believe that the care being delivered was not of the highest quality. However, they would likely respond with some level of distrust, possibly resulting in an incomplete information exchange and a less-than-optimal response to treatment.

The interactional and conceptional aspect of the experience and the inclusion of familiar service elements, as well as technical interventions, make the experience no less significant as a definer of quality.

Patients' experiences and perceptions of care are expressed and deliberated as patient satisfaction. Therefore, patient satisfaction is a valid outcome indicator of the quality of the entireness of care experienced [4,6,7].

Care or Cure?

Many disorders are self-limiting, meaning patients will recover with or without care. Care itself often does not cure. Some patients receive care designed to gain only a diagnosis (e.g., blood work, scans, biopsy), not a direct cure. For others, care is expected to result only in palliation of discomfort or temporary remission of symptoms. Some care is given to decry impairment, with no hope of a return to normal. End-of-life care doubtless is designed not to cure but to minimize discomfort and maximize the transitory quality of life of the patient, with death (not cure) the inevitable fade. Care for other patients does result in an intended and ostensibly permanent remission of disease, dysfunction, or symptoms.

This is the pure manifestation of cure and the ideal but frequently unrealized goal of care. No one—no hospital, no physician—can guarantee cure. The medical problem (e.g., infection, impairment, and organ failure), the patient's age, condition, life style, habits, personality, and support systems all can affect the ultimate outcome. But the hospital can guarantee care. Care includes technical intervention, empathy, information, and concern for the patient's emotional and physical comfort. Care is totally within the hospital's control [8,9].

If patients are highly satisfied with care in the broadest sense, then the most manageable part of the hospital's mission is achieved.

If a hospital's patients are dissatisfied with care, then that care is of lower quality, regardless of subsequent technical outcome [8,9].

The Link to Quality

Quality is defined as an immanent and remarkable attribute of a product or service. There is strong connection between patient satisfaction and overall quality of care, and high correlation between the patients' evaluations of the technical quality of their care and clinical experts' judgments of this same care. The patients' and physicians' ratings of hospital quality are highly connected and closely linked to patient satisfaction.

Common measures of quality are still structural measures - The condition of physical structure, floor space per bed, facilities for emergency power and lighting in operating rooms, inspection and cleaning of air intake sources, facilities for disposal of infectious waste, fire control and many more [10,11].

Many researchers also believe that patients are quite capable of judging the technical quality of care. This judgment is a very personal one, based on awareness of care being responsive to patients' individual needs rather than to any universal code of standards. When these individual needs are detected as being met, better care results. Others remark that lower care results when health professionals lack full control of their clinical areas or cannot communicate effectively and compassionately. In short, when patients perceive motives, communication, empathy, and clinical judgment positively, they will respond more positively to care. This includes physical and behavioral responses to care, not just emotional or estimational responses. Patient satisfaction is not only an indicator of the quality of care but a constituent of quality care as well. When patients are more satisfied, four things occur regarding trust, stress, safety, and the placebo effect [12,13,14,15].

Quality assessment

Effectiveness; Is the degree to which the care aimed or received has accomplished or can be expected to achieve, the greatest advancement in health possible now, given the patient's condition and the current state of science and technology of healthcare.

Efficiency; Is reflected as a ratio of actual or expected improvement in health to the cost of care responsible for these improvements. Thus, efficiency can be advanced by either improving care, reducing cost or both.

Optimality; Is a ratio of the effects of care on health or the financial benefits of these, or of the financial benefits of these effects to the cost of care.

Acceptability- depends on following factors:

- ❖ Accessibility
- ❖ The patient-practitioner relationship
- ❖ Amenities
- ❖ Patient preference as to the effect of care
- ❖ Patient preference as to the cost of care.

Legitimacy; Means compliance to social preference as reflected in ethical principles, values, norms, laws and regulations.

Equity- Is the principle of equity or justice in the distribution of care and of its benefit among the members of its population [12-15].

Trust Enhancement

Enhanced trust results in greater compliance as well as a greater tolerance of awkward or frightening procedures. The association between interaction skills (e.g., information giving and taking, empathy) and compliance are well recognized. Physicians generally are not fortunate at correctly identifying their compliant and noncompliant patients, most of times. Patients do not telegraph compliance. They do not usually voice complaints or question judgments on the spot, either. If patients not trust in the care, then medical management will be more difficult and likely less effective. There can be more complaints about discomfort or fear [12-15].

Importance of Communication

Physician communication or the lack of it, is probably one of the most important factors for patient noncompliance. Mayo Clinic found:

➢ 72% of patients were unable to list medications that they take.

> ➤ 58% of patients were unable to recite their own diagnosis.
> ➤ Inadequate communication between physicians, as well as between physicians and patients, is a major contributing factor for patient's re- admission [16].

Stress Reduction

The nursing care attribute showed the strongest influence on patient satisfaction, followed by staff care [17].

When the nurse puts a patient at ease, there is less stress, more relaxation of muscles, and an easier stick. Greater satisfaction means lower stress and less likelihood of complications. Stress reduction via empathetic interaction is clearly a vital factor. With increased stress, medical outcomes may be less satisfactory and higher costs are aroused because of complications [13].

The Placebo Effect

"Placebo" is Latin for "I please." estimates that, on average, 30 percent of any cure is a result of the placebo effect. This effect is emphatically not produced by the procedure itself (i.e., the pill or technical intervention).

Every intervention in the clinical setting has a placebo effect by affecting the patient's perception of care. Information, interaction, perceived motives and attitudes of caregivers, concern for physical comfort, decor, symbols, machinery, medications, treatments, every experience hand out to the intervention. All of these can have an effect on the patient's perception of the quality and efficiency of care while that care is being given, not just after discharge.

Physician enthusiasm, for example, can affect a patient's response to treatment, so can a confident attitude. One study of patients presenting with vague symptoms scripted doctors to use two different interactions. Doctors told one group of patients, "I don't know what's the matter with you." Patients in the other group were given a clear but benign diagnosis, such as duodenal inflammation, and were told that they needed no further treatment. Two weeks later, 39 percent of the first group reported feeling better, while sixty-four percent of the second group, which were told a definite diagnosis and prognosis, reported feeling better [18].

Safety and Satisfaction

Yet another advantage of high patient satisfaction is the likelihood of reduced errors. This takes several forms. First, if patients are more satisfied with general care, then they are likely to be more trusting, less stressed, less apprehensive by staff, and more cooperative during any specific aspect of care. This means that they will be more likely to ask questions and show concerns, especially if they feel something is not right. Information yields trust and should increase patients' responsibility for their own care [19].

In a Press Ganey study of 564,000 patients (Wolosin 2004), a number of informational issues were examined for their correlation with the hospital's concern for the patient's safety and security. Positive and highly statistically significant correlations were found between patient perceptions of their safety and the type and quality of information given during their stay. These issues involved nurses keeping the patient informed, explanations about what would happen during tests and treatments, information given to the family, and how well the physician kept the patient informed about what was going on.

Patients' perceptions of their safety in the hospital can be positively enhanced when staff make expressions or statements with obvious references to safety. When the nurse washes his hands with an antiseptic wipe in front of the patient or says, "we're checking the ID number on your wrist band to make sure we're giving you the right medicine," he is clearly showing the hospital's concern for the patient's safety [19,20].

In sum, when patients are more satisfied, medical management and outcome are enhanced. Patient satisfaction and real quality of care are not distinct phenomena. When your patients are more satisfied, they really are getting better care. Thus, when you measure patient satisfaction, you really are measuring your overall quality of care. Quality of care is defined by its effect on patients, not on its being acknowledged as such by professional experts.

Patients act on what they think or believe. If they think your institution is high in quality, then they will respond as though it is, regardless of the basis of their judgment [19,20].

Action for Satisfaction

Inform staff at all levels about the relation between patient satisfaction and the quality of care. This link is not intuitive. Staff must be recognized that the connection is direct (e.g., satisfaction and stress, compliance, information exchange) as well as indirect (e.g., a more satisfying general experience for the patient).

Patient satisfaction is assessed by a survey whose scores reflect staff performance as well as patient perspectives of the care delivered. Educate staff about the connection of the specific survey questions and specific aspects of care [19,21].

The link to Employee Satisfaction

That patient satisfaction is also a factor in staff satisfaction (and vice versa) is an added bonus, and depict a strong connection between employee satisfaction and patient intent to return to or recommend the hospital. In 2005, Press Ganey confirmed these findings in the largest study of its kind to date, examining the link between inpatient and employee satisfaction in 111 hospitals nationwide (in US). A key result of staff satisfaction is reduced turnover. In one medical center, reports that nursing staff turnover dropped from 16 percent to 11 percent as patient satisfaction made significant gains. In another health center they saw employee turnover drop from 24 percent to 18 percent (a 25 percent reduction) over the two-year period in which their satisfaction scores increased considerably [19,21]. Impacted by increased staff satisfaction, turnover reductions of this magnitude can mean significant savings through lower engagement and training costs.

Like the connection between satisfaction and quality of care, the patient/staff satisfaction relation is natural. The linkage is not quite direct, however. Administrators and policy can act as filters—or catalysts. When staff are empowered and thanked for behaviors and strategies that affect patient satisfaction, both staff and patient satisfaction will likely move upward. If patient satisfaction survey scores become a club with which to intimidate staff, and if staff are not rewarded for precisely addressing recognizable satisfaction issues, then both patients and staff may find less to endorse about your institution. If patient satisfaction is high, then staff will feel more content in their work and actualize the hospital's mission motivated way. High staff satisfaction is also a marker that staff feel enabled and supported by management in performing their personal missions of good patient care. The end result is more than mere job approval, of course. When provider satisfaction is elevated, the result is better medical treatment as well as personal care [19,21].

The link to Physician Satisfaction

Physician loyalty to the hospital can never be taken for granted.

A 2004 Press Ganey study of 11,000 physicians at 73 hospitals nationwide examined physician satisfaction with a range of hospital characteristics (Wolosin 2004). Among the most important supporters to their satisfaction were perceived quality of the hospital and care delivered, especially how well the institutional organization and the staff facilitated the physicians' ability to deliver quality care. When physicians are more satisfied, a smooth flow of information and technical events as well as a tighter coordination of care, is expressed. Patients can feel this through the care itself and their physician's comments, tone, and attitude.

As with the relationship between patient and employee satisfaction, the high linkage between patient and physician satisfaction with the hospital is not surprising.

A 2005 Press Ganey study in 94 hospitals nationwide demonstrated a strong, statistically significant correlation between patient and physician satisfaction with the hospital.

Physicians are affected by patient satisfaction both directly and indirectly. As indicated earlier, satisfied patients are more likely to be cooperative, informative, and synergetic. This makes the physician's job easier and can have a positive impact on outcome. More indirectly, physicians are aware of the hospital's quality initiatives and patient satisfaction programs, if any. Physicians in hospitals that put significant activity into building a patient satisfaction culture and publicizing their successes are more likely to be susceptible to patients' perceptions of care.

In hospitals with greater patient satisfaction, physicians feel more positive about their own efforts, their mission, and about the whole institution [19,21].

The correlation between case manager performance rating with global satisfaction is consistent with evidence indicating that provider behavior, including physician and nurse communication, is highly associated with patients' ratings of care. This finding has valuable impact for PCMHs (patient-centered medical home) that feature team-based care with nurse case managers because it indicates that case managers may affects patients' experiences in an ambulatory setting. Ambulatory practices may consider dedicating reserves to enhancing the communication and quality of care delivered by their case managers to improve the patient experience [22,23].

The second finding of the study was the relation between case manager performance rating and subsequent emergency department use.

Three possible mechanisms explain this finding.

> The first mechanism relates to attributes of a case manager. A higher quality case manager may be better equipped to avert diagnose and address problems, thereby decreasing following acute care needs.
> A second mechanism may be expressed by the relationship of the case manager and patient. A patient with greater trust in and a stronger connection with his or her case manager may be more likely to consult the case manager when problems emerge and adhere to the treatment plan and less likely to go to the emergency department.
> The third mechanism may be reflected by specific patient characteristics, such as patient activation, which may be individually associated with higher ratings of care as well as reduced acute care use. In addition to activation, other patient-side factors may separately affect care ratings and health care utilization, including mental health and substance abuse disorders, health literacy, and the degree of social support in the home.

These three mechanisms represent valuable areas for future investigation.

A final and unexpected finding in this study was the variability in overall satisfaction over time. Except for patient perceptions of access to care, the introduction of the PCMH has not significantly changed patient ratings of care. The discrepancy of this finding may be related to a change in patient selection for the case manager intervention over time rather than reflecting a true decline in satisfaction with care. Initial phases of the Proven Health Navigator at Geisinger targeted case manager services to the high risk patients and extended these services to more patients over time. Although sicker patients typically report lower ratings of care, it may be that sicker patients in a PCMH benefit most from a case manager intervention and are therefore more likely to report higher ratings of their case manager's performance [22,23].

Patient expectations

The concept of meeting patients' expectations for treatment is fundamental in their perception of satisfaction. Patients who consider their expectations for surgery were not met also reported less improvement when measured by functional outcome parameters. In a prospective study done by Albert Yee and colloquies [24], on 155 patient undergoing posterior lumbar spinal surgery for degenerative conditions. On follow up of 143 remaining patients were assessed with questionnaires (SF-36 and Oswestry Disability Index) preoperatively and six months (decompressions only) and one year (lumbar fusions) after surgery. They found that overall patient satisfaction with surgery as quantified in the postoperative questionnaire was 81%, (116 of 143). In 19% (27 of 143 patients) of patients, surgery did not meet overall expectations. Of these 27 patients, there were two cases of pseudarthroses, one case of pedicle screw misplacement, and three additional cases in which medical comorbidities were believed to be contributing factors.

For the 21 of 27 patients whose expectations for surgery were not met and no other poor prognostic factor could be identified, they observed lower reported preoperative SF-36 general health, vitality domain scores, and mean Mental Component scores (0.01, and 0.04, respectively).

Patients in whom expectations were not met also reported less improvement in SF-36 and Oswestry scores when compared with patients in whom expectations were met. Patients were likely to be less satisfied if they had prior lumbar surgery and were involved with workers' compensation or litigation. They also were more likely to undergo additional spinal surgery.

Even if the clinical expectations were met, some patients were still dissatisfied. Patients with spinal stenosis seem to have more unrealistic expectations than patients with disc herniation [24,25,26]

II

AIDET

The importance of keywords

AIDET and professionalism

A	I	D	E	T
Announce	Introduce	Duration	Explain	Thank you
Safety & respect	Decrease anxiety	Increase compliance	Quality	Patient loyalty

Table 1: AIDET scripting model.

AIDET is a standardized way of behaving, a habit shared by all members of the team. Professionalism is putting your client(s) ahead of you. Making a habit of using AIDET is one way of putting your client(s) first and is consistent with professional behavior.

The most valuable determinant of clinician global satisfaction is the doctor-patient relationship. The most common cause of malpractice suits is failed communication with the patients and their families. We have to explore ways that better communication will lead to fewer malpractice claims and allow healthcare organizations to reduce litigation costs [27,28].

For every customer (patient) that complains, there are 20 dissatisfied customers do not. Of those dissatisfied customers who do not complain, 90% do not return. The average wronged customer will tell 25 others. It is ten times more expensive to recruit new patients than to keep old ones. An evidence-based practice for communicating with patients, families and staff.

A survey was designed in July of 2007 to be used by Studer Group AIDET product for evaluation of partners and non-partners, who had purchased the AIDET video series during the time period of November 2005 to April 2007.

Baseline data were collected and results were measured over a 6- month time period after initial implementation began [28].

The impact on physician satisfaction; within 12 months of implementing AIDET, physician satisfaction went from the 53rd percentile to the 93rd percentile. AIDET was a large contributing factor in this change of physician perspective."

The importance of keywords

Using keywords or phrases in AIDET reflects an understanding of human behavior, the need to alleviate fears and anxiety, and the need to build trust. The patient has the right to know who is treating them. Because greetings are one way to ensure proper identification of patients, they may well be considered a substantial component of patient safety. It's all about building connection. Connection builds trust. Trust builds patient compliance. Compliance builds better health for our patients. And that's the real picture [28,29].

Consider the power of keywords and phrases such as "please, thank you, excuse me or I'm sorry. Use keywords & phrases repetitively in AIDET! These are powerful, positive words & phrases such as concern, comfort, thorough, careful, expert, communicate, informed, we're on the same team, protection, your privacy, etc. Avoid negative words & avoid blaming others—choose your words carefully, both verbal & written!

All these will build up patient confidence and satisfaction, like the equation below;

Decreased Anxiety	+	Increased Compliance	=	Improved clinical outcomes & Increased patient & physician satisfaction

A: Acknowledge; Safety and respect

Key Message: All of you are important... Translated to the patient in many ways like;

➤ Eye contact
➤ Acknowledge everyone in the room & determine their names & relationships
➤ Shake hands with the whole
➤ Ensure you're speaking with the appropriate patient

Smile, look like you love what you are doing [28,29].

I: Introduce; Decrease anxiety, building trust to increase compliance

Key Message: Your health team is competent... Expressed by identifying;

➤ Name of the patient
➤ Name and specialty ; your role in the team
➤ Your years of experience & credentials
➤ Wear name on badge or coat
➤ Hand out your card

Other information to manage up [28,29].

D: Duration;

Key Message: I anticipate your concerns

- How long before the doctor will see the patient? (requires physician communication with the nurse and staff)
- How long will the appointment/hospitalization be?
- How long will the test, procedure, visit, appointment actually take?
- How long will it take to get the results?
- When is our next meeting?

Key words & phrases: (We have a reputation for being very THOROUGH), (We first need to review all the tests very CAREFULLY) [28,29].

E: Explanation.... Quality

Key Message: We will decide on a plan together.

The key driver for patient satisfaction is the quality and clarity of information that patients receive from physicians.

During a 20-minute encounter, physicians self-report spending 9 minutes "providing information", while the reality is the physicians spent only1.5 minutes. So it's vital to listen to the patient by;

- Sit down (side of bed/chair)
- Active listening
- Eye contact
- Empathy
- Avoid appearing impatient
- Don't shake or tap
- Don't observe time discreetly

Explain...

> Use language that patients can understand
> Use key words & phrases like (We are CONCERNED, so we would like to order), (For your COMFORT), (To PROTECT your RIVACY), (I want to keep you INFORMED), and (We CARE about PROTECTING you from having another event).
> Do you need more explanation? [28,30].

T: Thank You, Patient loyalty

Key Message: We feel fortunate to have had the opportunity to care for you / work with you.

> Thank you for:
> Choosing our clinic / hospital / OU Medicine
> Waiting / your patience
> Helping us with this project
> What other questions do you have?
> Is there anything else I can do for you?
> Is there anything else we could have done to make your experience better? [28,30].

Post Discharge Phone Calls

Discharge phone calls are an effective method to gain patient loyalty, enhance quality of care, clinical outcomes and develop a reputation of excellence in the community when steadily completed. Discharge phone calls are a key element in the saving lives back up. Discharge telephone calls provide invaluable opportunities to avoid adverse events, improve quality of care, and increase patient satisfaction.

Evidence suggests that a post-discharge telephone call to patients may help diminish medication errors and hospital readmission. Discharge phone calls close the gap on continuity of care for the patient and family.

You have a 90 percent chance of keeping a patient if you call within 48 hours of discharge and do something (like apologize) to make the patient's experience better.

If you wait longer than a week, you have a 10 percent chance you'll lose 10 other patients through word of mouth [31-34].

In a study by Riegel and colloquies, they found that follow-up telephone calls considerably decreased the average number of hospital days over six month time and readmission rate at six months in the call group, as well as increased patient satisfaction [35].

Nurse Hourly Rounding

Rationale:

- Actively engages patients and families
- Trust building
- Anxiety reduction
- Call light reduction
- Decreases nurse stress
- Decreases patient uncertainty

Hourly rounding has an excellent influence on patient perception and quality of care;

- Hourly rounding adequately decreases call lights by 37.8%
- Decreases falls by 50%
- Decreases hospital-acquired decubiti by 14%
- Enhances patient perception by 12 mean points [36,37,38]

Leader Rounding

Leader rounding for outcomes is the first key to success. The point of rounding for outcomes is;

- To fix systems, remove barriers, model behavior, and find staff who is worthy to be rewarded and recognized.
- To be enrolled in the very important process of building an emotional bank account with staff.

➤ Senior leader rounds give leaders an opportunity to express their appreciation to the patients who have chosen the hospital for care.

Merits of Leader Rounding on Patients

➤ Increase patients satisfaction by an average 59 percentile, patients who are visited by a nurse leader during their hospital stay are more likely to give top box ratings across all HCAHPS (Hospital Consumer Assessment of Healthcare Providers and Systems) measures.
➤ Decrease patient complaints by 66%.
➤ Reduce Emergency Department LWOT (leaving without treatment) from 4.5% to 2%.

Merits of Leader Rounding on Staff

➤ Improved employee satisfaction from 10th to 75th percentile
➤ Reduce voluntary/non voluntary turnover from 11.2% to 6.1%
➤ Improve retention from 82.5% to 87.2%
➤ Decrease vacancy rate from 7% to 2% [34, 39-41].

III

Patient Reported Outcome

Measuring relevant outcomes in a timely manner is a priority in a health care system progressively focused on the delivery of high-value care. Most quality measures focus on care processes or definitive outcomes such as survival; until recently, there has been less emphasis on quantitative measurements of functional outcomes, symptoms, and quality of life [44,45].

Symptom management is a keystone of clinical care, especially for patients with chronic conditions. Yet patients' symptoms and physical deterioration go unnoticed by health care providers as much as half the time, specifically between clinic visits. As a result, we miss opportunities to intervene and alleviate suffering. Moreover, incomplete documentation of this information in the electronic health record (EHR) restricts our ability to understand key patient outcomes when we aggregate EHR data for comparative effectiveness research or quality-of care assessments. Recent advances in technology and survey methods provide a potential solution in the form of patient-reported outcomes (PROs) with standardized questionnaires, it is one way of getting this information, recorded electronically, the questionnaires completed by patients at or between visits over the internet or on a smart device, with data transmitted into the EHR. Clinicians can receive automated notifications about alarming symptoms or functional issues, such as severe dyspnea or reduced physical activity in an outpatient with heart failure. They can review longitudinal PRO reports at visits and manipulate that information into their EHR notes as a part of the review of systems. It's believed that this approach can positively impact patients' quality of life, boost patient–doctor communication, decrease emergency department use, and lengthen survival, PROs can also play a role in shared decision making, and may enhance physician satisfaction in addition to improve patient care. Many organizations have successfully enrolled systematic PRO collection into routine clinical care. Partners HealthCare, a large multihospital system in Boston, introduced PROs system-wide in 2012 and has since collected more than 1.2 million PRO scores in 75 clinics across 21 specialties, including urology, orthopedics, psychiatry, and primary care. As comfort with PROs has grown, feedback has increasingly maintained that clinicians find collecting PROs to be beneficial rather than inconvenient. Evidence from experienced users suggests PRO collection may even enhance physician satisfaction and prevent burnout. Many aspects of patient care may be compromised by burnout. Physicians who have burnout are more likely to report making recent medical errors, score lower on instruments measuring empathy, and plan to retire early and have higher job dissatisfaction, which has been associated with lowered patient satisfaction with medical care and patient adherence to treatment plans [44-47].

Moreover, PROs can promote workflow efficiency and save time when they're used regularly. PROs can improve relationships between physicians and patients by permitting providers to better understand patients' symptoms. For example, collecting PROs gave spine surgeons a quantitative measure of the extent to which patients were agonizing to cope with their postsurgical pain. Surgeons could then take appropriate action, such as referring certain patients to a behavioral pain psychologist. PROs also gave healthcare providers a more data driven understanding of post-procedure recovery profiles. The information gathered from these assessments often differed from physicians' long-held assumptions and helped them better collaborate with patients during the recovery process. PROs can also enhance shared decision making. Both the physician and the patient felt better about the process and outcome of their PRO-facilitated conversation [44-48].

Moreover, PROs can improve workflow efficiency and save time when they're used regularly. One primary care physician noted that using electronic surveys that included a screening questionnaire, risk assessments, and a review of systems enabled her to "be a doctor again." Because patients had already answered screening questions electronically while in her clinic's waiting room, she was no longer forced to navigate through verbal checklists during visits. Instead, she examined and communicated, focusing on the issues that most required her attention. She saved about 10 minutes on each annual physical, and for the first time in years, her practice ran on schedule. Other thing is the PROs have improved conversations that might not otherwise have taken place by allowing sensitive issues to be raised in systematic ways, like symptoms related to sexual dysfunction, incontinence, and rectal bleeding, or spouse maltreatment or negligence and domestic abuse [48-50].

In spite of all above, examination of PROs has not become a widely integral part of routine care delivery. A common thread in the PRO initiatives implemented to date is that they originated with clinician champions with support from institutional leadership. All these institutions systematically evaluated their patients' and clinicians' needs to inform the development of technology-driven approaches for integrated patients' voices into routine care delivery. Despite these challenges, we believe PROs have the potential to reengage patients and physicians in the care delivery process. Far from being only a strategy to satisfy payers or prove the value of certain technologies, PROs could help sustain the size and spirit of the physician workforce, providing a much-needed path to a stronger health care system [50-52].

Beyond clinical care, systematically collected PRO data can be collected and linked to other electronic health record EHR information to support analyses of effectiveness (e.g., which of various interventions controls back pain best?), examinations of quality of care (e.g., do different providers or practices manage post-chemotherapy nausea differently?), and pharmaco-vigilance (e.g., is a particular drug associated with unexpected symptoms?). Indeed, there is enlarging national interest in controlling patient-reported data in all these areas. There is adequate scientific belief and understanding of administration methods to extend collection of PRO data in clinical care. Doing so could turn the fluency about the "patient-centered care" into a reality [53].

Greater fulfillment of expectations will lead to greater postoperative satisfaction and associate with enhanced functional outcomes in patients undergoing cervical and lumbar spine surgeries. This dictates the value of preoperative expectations which should be taken seriously to obtain an informed choice on the basis of patient's preferences.

There are only few available studies investigating the correlation between PROs and satisfaction in spine surgery. A recent study investigating predictors for anterior cervical spine surgery reported that VAS neck pain and NDI were valid predictors for satisfaction after 2 and 5 years [17,54, 55].

The outcome of treatment was overall, the most salient predictor followed by nursing kindness as the second most important component [56].

Patient reported satisfaction and its impact on outcomes in spinal surgery

Satisfaction plays an important role in patient care as discontented patients are less likely to attend follow-up appointments as well as comply with treatment plans. While the exact link remains unclear, higher patient satisfaction has been associated with lower costs, mortality rates and minor complication rates [57].

Like many surgeries, spine surgery is generally performed to relieve and reduce patient symptomatology. These procedures are often performed electively and thus patients make their decisions to undergo surgical intervention based on personal expectations and goals. A critical role of the healthcare provider in these circumstances is to assess the patient's understanding of their condition such that they can make an informed decision. Akhila Sure and colloquies [58] had perform a study is to review the literatures in regards to patient satisfaction after undergoing spine surgery in order to help elucidate the significance of patient satisfaction. They found factors that have been shown to positively correlate with post-operative patient satisfaction scores include: greater pre-operative self-estimated walking distance, type of procedure performed, region of the spine being operated upon, expectation to return to work, if the surgeon recommended the operative intervention, lower pre-operative expectations, and time spent by the healthcare provider with the patient. Moreover, subjective measures such as achievement of expectations, higher perceived and actual improvement in overall function, and greater reduction in pain have also been correlated with higher patient satisfaction [57,58].

Sigmundsson et al. found that a history of previous spine surgery, smoking, unemployment, back pain exceeding 1 year, and a symptom profile predominated by back pain to be associated with decreased patient satisfaction after spine surgery, of which prior spine surgery decreased the odds of satisfaction the most [59].

The difference between a patient's pre-operative expectation and the actual postoperative outcomes, in particular, can be a significant predictor of patient satisfaction in spine surgery. This gap was first coined the "Expectation-Actuality Discrepancy" (EAD) by Mannion et al. which suggested that a main factor driving patient satisfaction is the fulfillment of expectations. A small E-AD, signifying that more realistic patient expectations prior to spine surgery tend to leave patients more satisfied with their procedure afterwards. A specific expectation that patients hold may influence their level of satisfaction. Patients who held realistic expectations concerning pain and physical recovery enjoyed a greater chance of being satisfied [60].

Likewise, higher pre-operative expectations were found to be associated with lower satisfaction despite improved overall functional outcomes. Mancuso et al. examined expectations and satisfaction following lumbar and cervical spine surgery over 2 years. His study found that 90% of lumbar patients and 91% of cervical patients had some amount of their expectations met post-operatively, and that loftier baseline expectations generally led to fewer fulfillments of those expectations following their procedure [61].

Now, attention to PROs is growing as part of routine clinical practice, spurred in part by provisions in the healthcare institutions, and the increasing presence of electronic formats or collecting and storing survey data is fueling the ability to collect PROs.

PROs might include information about which outcomes matter most to patients as well as actual measures o symptoms, functional status, or quality of life. Collection of such outcomes is especially relevant to conditions involving longitudinal care such as cancer, heart disease, mental illness, or arthritis. There is growing interest in developing standardized instruments or collecting PRO-performance measures has been issued [57,58,62].

Hospitalists can better meet patients individualized needs by taking the following steps:

> Acquire and maintain communication skills and cultural competency.
> Identify who the patient does and does not want involved in his or her care, including his or her surrogate decision maker.
> Communicate in the patient's native language.
> Encourage and empower family presence.
> Confirm that the patient-family understand information presented to them, via techniques such as "Ask-Tell-Ask," and decision aids to illustrate difficult concepts (such as a videotape or printed algorithms) [57, 58,62].

Involving patients in system design

Improved coordination of care or a patient can help but more broadly, the concept of patient-centered care extends beyond the approach to the individual patient, and includes as a tenet that patients have a voice in the design of the care delivery system itself. Now hospitals do involve patients in operational steps, either by creating positions for patients or family members on existing hospital committees, and/or creating a separate "Patient/Family Advisory Council" (PFAC) function. In fact the presence of a PFAC is now advanced by regulation in some states. An institution may have a single PFAC or multiple PFACs based on a desire or specific patient involvement in discreet service lines. A role or patient/ family collaboration has been described or a variety of administrative procedures, including strategic planning, facility redesign, research oversight, ethics, care coordination, education, finance, credentialing, leadership search, information technology, process improvement, patient safety, service excellence, and personnel practices [58,62].

Patient experience of care

In 2011, the Centers for Medicare & Medicaid Services (CMS) established Hospital Value-Based Purchasing (HVBP), a new hospital reimbursement system designed to shift payment models away from the traditional fee-for-service system and toward rewarding health care quality. Under HVBP, CMS withholds 2% of reimbursement from all hospitals, which are then redistributed from low-performing to high-performing hospitals based on their total performance score (TPS) [63].

Patient experience accounts for 25% of a hospital's TPS and is composed of 9 dimensions derived from the Hospital Consumer Assessment of Healthcare Providers and Systems (HCAHPS) survey. The percentage of patients who provide the highest possible HCAHPS response, termed a "top-box" response, for each branch is used to estimate an institution's TPS. As the patient experience of care begins to play a more important role in assessing the quality of care, it is essential to identify which elements of hospital experience are most strongly associated with a highly satisfying overall patient experience. The need to identify the determinants of patient satisfaction is particularly acute for common and costly procedures, which have the largest potential impact on hospital reimbursement [64].

In a retrospective study done by Jay M. Levin and colloquies [65] of HCAHPS (Hospital Consumer Assessment of Healthcare Providers and Systems) surveys collected from patients who underwent lumbar spine surgery aims to identify the individual components of patient experience that are most strongly associated with a highly satisfying overall hospital experience during lumbar spine surgery. In our study, a top-box response to the Overall Hospital Rating (OHR) component of the HCAHPS survey—the only dimension of the survey that assesses the overall experience and is used in HVBP calculations— was used to measure the patients' overall experience in the hospital.

The result of these surveys, are 80.1% recorded a top-box OHR, thus composing the satisfied group. The overall health status was the only variable found to be a significant predictor of overall satisfaction with the hospital experience. Diminishing overall health status was observed to be a negative predictor of overall satisfaction. The individual survey items that were associated with the greatest increased odds of predictors of overall satisfaction were as in the following:

> Hospital staff always did everything they could to help with pain
> Nurses were always courteous and respectful
> Nurses always listened carefully
> Medication side effects were always explained
> Personal and family preferences were always taken into account
> Doctors were always courteous and respectful
> Patient room and bathroom were always kept clean
> Patient had a good understanding of what he/she was responsible for in managing health when leaving the hospital
> Pain was always well controlled

This study therefore analyzed HCAHPS responses from lumbar spine surgery patients to determine the most influential predictors of overall satisfaction in this population. They found that the two strongest predictors of overall satisfaction were the patient perception that the staff always did everything they could to help with pain, and that nurses were always respectful and courteous [65].

Providing a satisfying inpatient experience may be under direct control of the hospital and its staff, and can therefore become a guaranteed positive outcome of spine surgery from the patient perspective, especially once the key drivers of satisfaction are explained. This is especially critical because, on the contrary, surgical outcomes are sometimes uncertain in spine surgery [66].

Waiting time

The clinical ambulatory patient experience is largely impacted by time spent waiting for provider care. Not only are records regarding the likelihood to recommend and the overall satisfaction with the experience negatively impacted by longer wait times, but increased wait times also affect perceptions of information, instructions, and the overall treatment provided by physicians and other caregivers. Longer wait times are negatively associated with clinical provider scores of patient satisfaction, results indicated that every aspect of patient experience, specifically confidence in the care provider and perceived quality of care, linked negatively with longer wait times [67-71].

Successful Strategies for Waiting Rooms

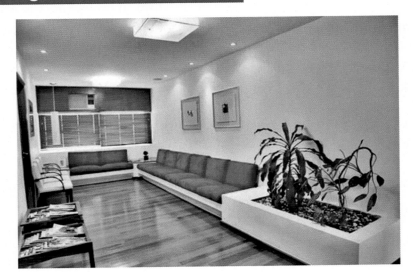

The experience of waiting is an integral component of overall patient satisfaction. The ideal waiting area should provide conversational groupings, charging stations for mobile devices, places to watch TV, and tables between or near seating to hold food and drink. To improve the familiarity, waiting room furniture should fit the bodies of the people who use it, including children and high-weight individuals. Furnishings should adjust different postures, behaviors, and levels of privacy. Thoughtful space planning is another tool that can reduce anxiety during the wait. Updated lining up models can also improve patient perceptions of waiting time [67-71].

Pain management

Adequate pain management promotes earlier mobility and decreases the complications of ileus, urinary retention, and myocardial infarction. Sleep deprivation, which can increase postoperative fatigue, resulting in decreased mobility, is also reduced, as are pulmonary complications, and an aggravated catabolic hormonal response to injury. When physiological complications are better controlled, patients and their families are better able to respond to stress and to cope with the patient's situation. Additional gains of adequate pain management include decreased length of stay, lower readmission rates, earlier overall recovery, improved quality of life, increased productivity, and decreased costs for patients and the health care system, in other words improved patient outcomes and increased patient satisfaction [72,73]. The clinical practice guidelines of the American Pain Society recommend that patients and their families receive pain education during the pre-surgical visit that includes an explanation of the surgical procedure; the expected postoperative routine; the interventions and options for pain relief, including available pain medication; and the need for progressive increased mobility [72-74]. Adequate education and proper treatment of postoperative pain can also impact a positive emotional outcomes for patients, such as a decrease in anxiety and depression, an increase in coping skills, a greater sense of individual control, and a boost in a sense of well-being [72-76].

A thorough pain history and shared goal setting are critical elements of effective pain management that leads to beneficial outcomes.

Proper pain education and precise treatment of postoperative pain can result in positive emotional outcomes.

Although research and advanced treatments in improved practice protocols have documented progressive improvements in management of acute and postoperative pain, little awareness of the effectiveness of best practices persists. Improved interventions can enhance patients' attitudes to and perceptions of pain. What a patient believes and understands about pain is critical in influencing the patient's reaction to the pain therapy provided. Use of interdisciplinary pain teams can lead to improvements in patients' pain management, pain education, outcomes, and satisfaction [72-76].

During the past two decades, professional associations, accrediting bodies, and payers have made post-surgical pain treatment a high priority. A survey was conducted by Tong J Gan [77] and colloquies included a random sample of US adults who had undergone surgery within 5 years from the survey date. Participants were asked about their concerns before surgery, severity of perioperative pain, pain treatments, perceptions about post-surgical pain and pain medications, and satisfaction with treatments they received, to assess patient perceptions and characterize patient experiences/levels of satisfaction with post-surgical pain management. Of the 300 participants, ~86% experienced pain after surgery; of these, 75% had moderate/extreme pain during the immediate post-surgical period, with 74% still experiencing these levels of pain after discharge.

Post-surgical pain was the most striking pre-surgical patient concern, and nearly half reported they had high/very high anxiety levels about pain before surgery. Approximately 88% received analgesic medications to manage pain; of these, 80% experienced adverse effects and 39% reported moderate/ severe pain even after receiving their first dose [77].

Non-pharmacologic approaches such as psychosocial support should be introduced to the patients. Proper guidance and information should be given to healthcare providers to improve the quality of patient care. Healthcare providers should adopt a sensitive approach in caring for patients' needs. The aim is to meet the needs of the patients who want to be pain free or to attain adequate relief of their pain for breakthrough pain [78].

Pain management programs that focus on patient-provider communication may succeed in helping patients better understand how hospital staff is working to diminish pain. In a national survey of 250 adults who underwent surgery, Apfelbaum et al. found that only two-thirds of patients were spoken to by a health care professional about their pain. If, as the current results suggest, communication improves inpatient pain management, then it is possible that patient satisfaction can improve without boosting an increased utilization of opioid analgesic medications [65,79].

The addition of a 5-minute massage treatment at the time of analgesic administration significantly increased patient satisfaction with pain management [Jane Miller] [80].

Family involvement

Patients prefer direct family involvement in their health care more often than what occurs in practice. Physicians can easily address this discrepancy by asking patients whether and in what way they would like others to be engaged in their health care [81,82].

In a study done by Sara Locatelli and colloquies, they found that patient and family engagement was addressed to be a key element of the design and accomplishment of patient centered care innovations. Moreover it offers a unique perspective and key understanding of Veterans' needs, and allow employees/providers to discover unexpected outcomes. Offering multiple engagement options maximizes patients and families involved and ensures feedback is approved from a variety of sources [83].

Family involvement is an integral dimension of patient-centered care. Evidence far indicates that the more active family members are in physician visits, the more highly satisfied patients are with their usual care provider and that patients also participate more actively in decision making. In a study done by Jennifer L. Wolff and colloquies, they found that patients companion facilitation of doctor understanding (by giving the doctor information about the patient's medical history or symptoms (e.g. 'she fell last week and bruised her arm') was significantly associated with both the patient and companion giving the doctor more medical information. Companions' facilitation of patient understanding was also associated with fewer questions by the doctor. Facilitation of doctor understanding was associated with greater patient biomedical information giving [84].

Empathy

Unfortunately, the trajectory of medicine's increasingly one-sided focus on science and technology over the humanities has created an ever-widening gap between physicians and patients, resulting in decreased trust and confidence in a relationship that needs and depends on it the most. A medicine practiced without a genuine and obligating awareness of what patients go through may fulfill its technical goals, but it is an empty medicine, or, at best, half a medicine [85].

Physician behavior was related to patients' ratings of satisfaction and perceived autonomy. When physicians were rated as more empathic by independent coders, patients reported a higher rate of "excellent" satisfaction than when physicians were rated as less empathic. Because empathy is defined as physicians understanding patients' perspectives, this might make patients feel more understood, and thus more satisfied. In one study, empathy in patient-physician encounters was related to patient behavior change. Another study showed that when physicians expressed compassion for as few as 40 seconds, patients felt better and less anxious [86,87].

In a study done by Kathryn I. Pollak and colloquies, to determine if physician use of specific motivation interviewing techniques increases patient satisfaction with the physician and perceived autonomy. They found patients whose physicians were rated as more empathetic had higher rates of high satisfaction than patients whose physicians were less empathetic. Patients whose physicians made any reflective statements had higher rates of high autonomy support than those whose physicians did not. Patient-physician communication is an integral component of high-quality care [88].

Patient's listening

- ❖ A patient's listening is motivated by a universal need:
  - ➢ The need for compassion
  - ➢ The need to be heard
  - ➢ The need to be recognized
- ❖ From a tone of voice or acknowledgment, the patient can readily hear if the white coat standing in front of him/her is someone who can care enough to listen [16,85].

Hospital length of stay

In a retrospective cohort study, to assess what factors impose to increased hospital LOS (length of stay) in patients who have had an ACDF, Paul M Arnold and his colloquies, extensively analyze the preoperative, intraoperative, and postoperative data of 108 consecutive patients to assign the prognostic factors for an increased LOS. They found the elements that contributed to increased LOS and their associated adjusted mean days were:

- ➢ Age ≥ 50 years of (2.5 ± 1.2 days).
- ➢ Female gender (2.3 ± 1.2 days).
- ➢ Cardiac complications, (3.5 ± 1.3 days); (hypertension and broadly defined cardiac or non-cardiac chest pain. Most complaints of chest pain were due to neck muscles pulling on the chest wall; no actual cardiac events occurred postoperatively as verified by cardiac work-up.
- ➢ Urinary complications (4.7 ± 1.3 days); (urinary retention, problems urinating after Foley removal.
- ➢ Pulmonary complications (5.3 ± 1.3 days); (decreased saturation, need for O2 and aggressive pulmonary toilet, exacerbation of asthma, respiratory failure, atelectasis, pneumonia) [89].

IV

The HCAHPS

Hospital Consumer Assessment of Healthcare Providers and Systems

Definition; A standardized survey tool to qualify the patient's perception of quality of care received during their experience while a patient at an acute-care hospital. Its importance as the patient perception of care will be publicly reported with other performance indicators on the hospital data unit. The information will be used to offer valuable details for improvement efforts as well as provide comparisons between hospitals to help consumers choose a hospital.

The patient's perception of a hospital performance is a reportable and real reflection of the hospital's reputation [90,91].

Overview

The HCAHPS (Hospital Consumer Assessment of Healthcare Providers and Systems) survey is the first national, standardized, publicly reported survey of patients' prospects about hospital care. HCAHPS is a 32-item survey instrument and data collection methodology for assessing patients' perceptions of their hospital experience. While many hospitals have gathered information on patient satisfaction for their own internal use, until HCAHPS there were no common metrics and no national standards for collecting and publicly sharing data regarding patient experience of care. Since 2008, HCAHPS has allowed valid comparisons to be made across hospitals locally, regionally and nationally (in the US).

Three wide goals have configured HCAHPS. First, the formulated survey and enforcement system produces information that allow objective and meaningful comparisons of hospitals on issues which are critical to patients and consumers. Second, public reporting of HCAHPS results provides new opportunities for hospitals to enhance quality of care. Third, public reporting leads to improve accountability in health care by strengthening transparency of the quality of hospital care provided in exchange for the public investment [90-92].

HCAHPS Development, Testing and Endorsement

Beginning in 2002, CMS (Centers for Medicare & Medicaid Services) partnered with the Agency for Healthcare Research and Quality (AHRQ), another agency in the Federal Department of Health and Human Services, to develop and test the HCAHPS Survey. AHRQ and its CAHPS Consortium accomplished a firm and multi-faceted scientific process, including a public call for framework, literature review, cognitive interviews, consumer focus groups, stakeholder effect, a three-state pilot test, extensive psychometric investigation, consumer testing, and multiple small-scale field measures. CMS provided three opportunities for the public to comment on HCAHPS and responded to over a thousand comments. The survey, its methodology and the results it provides are in the public domain [90-92].

HCAHPS Survey Content and Administration

The HCAHPS survey asks newly discharged patients about issues of their hospital encounter that they are uniquely concerned. The heart of the survey contains 21 items that ask "how often" or whether patients experienced a critical aspect of hospital care, rather than whether they were "satisfied" with their care. Also included in the survey are four screener items that direct patients to relevant questions, five items to adjust for the mix of patients across hospitals, and two items that support Congressionally-mandated reports. Hospitals may add supplemental issues after the primary HCAHPS items.

HCAHPS is accomplished to a random sample of adult inpatients between 48 hours and six weeks after discharge. Patients admitted in the medical, surgical and maternity care service lines are qualified for the survey; HCAHPS is not restricted to Medicare patients. Hospitals may use a qualified survey dispenser or collect their own HCAHPS information, if approved by CMS to do so. HCAHPS can be accomplished in four survey modes: Mail Only, Telephone Only, Mixed (mail with telephone follow-up), or Active Interactive Voice Response (IVR), each of which requires multiple attempts to contact patients. Hospitals should survey patients throughout each month of the year. IPPS (Inpatient Prospective Payment System) hospitals must achieve at least 300 completed surveys over four calendar quarters. HCAHPS is available in official English, Spanish, Chinese, Russian, Vietnamese, and Portuguese translations. The survey and its protocols for sampling, data collection, coding and submission can be found in the HCAHPS Quality Assurance Guidelines (QAG) manual located under the Quality Assurance section of the official HCAHPS Web site at http://hcahpsonline.org [90-92].

HCAHPS Measures

The HCAHPS survey involves 21 patient perspectives on care and patient rating items that comprise nine key topics: communication with doctors, communication with nurses, responsiveness of hospital staff, pain management, communication about medicines, discharge information, cleanliness of the hospital environment, quietness of the hospital environment, and transition of care. The survey also involves four screener questions and seven demographic issues, which are used for modifying the mix of patients through hospitals and for analytical benefits. The survey is 32 questions in length. Eleven HCAHPS measures (seven summary measures, two individual items and two global items) are currently publicly reported on the Hospital Compare Web site at https://www.medicare.gov/hospitalcompare. Each of the seven summaries, or composite, measures is constructed from two or three survey questions. Merging related questions into composites allows consumers to quickly review patient experience data and increases the statistical reliability of the measures. The seven composites summarize how well nurses and doctors communicate with patients, how responsive hospital staff are to patients' needs, how well hospital staff help patients manage pain, how well the staff communicates with patients about new medicines, whether key information is provided at discharge, and how well patients understand the type of care they need after leaving the hospital. The two individual items address the cleanliness and quietness of patients' rooms while the two global items capture patients' overall rating of the hospital and whether they would recommend it to family and friends. Survey response rates and the number of completed surveys are also publicly reported. There are three issues on the new correlation about pain structure measure, focus on correspondence between healthcare workers and patients about pain [90-94].

HCAHPS scores are configured and prepared for use at the hospital level for the comparison of hospitals to each other. CMS does not review or adopt the use of HCAHPS scores for comparisons within hospitals, such as comparison of HCAHPS scores associated with a particular ward, floor, individual staff member, etc. to others. Such comparisons are unreliable unless large sample sizes are collected at the ward, floor, or individual staff member level. In addition, since HCAHPS questions inform about wide spectrum of hospital staff (such as doctors in general and nurses in general rather than specific individuals), HCAHPS is not appropriate for comparing or assessing individual staff members. Using HCAHPS scores to compare or assess individual staff members is inappropriate and is strongly discouraged by CMS [90-95].

What do patients want from the healthcare provider?

Communication with doctors, communication with nurses, responsiveness of hospital staff, pain management, communication about medicines, discharge information, cleanliness of hospital environment, quietness of hospital environment, overall rating of hospital, and willingness to recommend the hospital, all these are the key issues for patients to trust the healthcare system.

How Will HCAHPS Reinforce Focus on Quality?

* Patient-Centered care is a quality indicator
* Quality no longer the domain of just the clinicians
* Gives a voice to the patient perception of safety
* Highlights communication issues/barriers
* Patient-centered care actively involves patients in their care
* More senior leaders are engaged and interested in delivering patient-centered care
* HCAHPS aligns with CEO's top issues [92,95].

Common Challenges

The most common HCAHPS concern is response rates. Nearly two out of three respondents encounter with this issue. Most depend on some manner of verbal, pre-discharge discussion with patients, followed up by phone and/or mail surveys with results split fairly evenly between the two. Among the themes measured in HCAHPS surveys, participants engage fairly uniformly. The most perplexing areas, however, are physician communication, staff responsiveness and transition of care. The latter is one of the newest HCAHPS measures, and it will take most hospitals some time to hardwire procedures that enhance those scores. There's a wide range of response when it comes to HCAHPS. In terms of a definitive solution to increase response rates or shifting emotion, the study didn't reveal a simple answer. In fact, simply reading the report for an easy answer to HCAHPS scores would be to miss the point [90,92,95].

Improving Response Rate Strategies

- ❖ Inform patients about the survey, mostly at discharge - Flyer or brochure - Posters, hospital website, announcements on waiting room television screens.
- ❖ Remind patients during discharge phone calls.
- ❖ Leader rounding – assess patient satisfaction during stay and/or remind of survey.
- ❖ Weekly or biweekly patient lists to vendors [92,95].

Overall HCAHPS Success strategies

- ❖ Culture; Standards of behavior - Teamwork – Accountability.
- ❖ Leadership practices; Leader visibility - Leadership development - Leader rounding with staff.
- ❖ HCAHPS Data Feedback; Share the information with staff and providers often - Provide opportunities for discussion and suggestions - Promote friendly competition.
- ❖ Staff Engagement; Consistent, intentional involvement in decision making and problem solving - Celebrations of performance improvement progress, rewards and recognition.
- ❖ Additional Strategies; Evaluations or pay for performance tied to HCAHPs - Hire for fit - Dedicated staff or committee -Staffing ratios [91].

Communication with Nurses

The nurse patient relationship regulates the tone of the care experience and has a tremendous effect on patient satisfaction since nursing spends the most time with patients. Based on 2007 HCAHPS and Press Ganey Survey data, Press Ganey identified "Nurse Communication" as the factor with the greatest impact on patients' overall ratings of their hospital experience. Survey questions that compress on the nurse patient relationship drive patient ratings of their overall experience. Quality of communication in nursing also has the highest effect on patients' likelihood to recommend the hospital [96].

Patient whiteboards are the most commonly reported effect measures concerning the nursing communication, followed by nurse bedside shift report, hourly rounding (discussed under "responsiveness of hospital staff"), scripting, and daily meetings. Other interventions not already addressed during overall HCAHPS performance are nurses rounding with physicians, multidisciplinary rounding, and mandatory scrub colors [91,92,96].

Key Strategies

- ❖ Patient whiteboards
- ❖ Nurse bedside shift report
- ❖ Data feedback and discussion
- ❖ Scripting
- ❖ Daily meetings
- ❖ Hourly rounding
- ❖ Leader rounding with patients
- ❖ Nurse engagement/ownership
- ❖ Mandatory scrub colors [91].

Communication with Physicians

Patients put greater emphasis on doctors' communication skills than their professional judgment or experience, and doctors failing in these areas are the primary concern that drives patients to shift.

How Do Patients Judge Quality?

- ❖ Did the physician listen?
- ❖ Did the physician express concern?
- ❖ Did the physician answer my questions?
- ❖ Did the physician care for me as a person, and not just a patient?
- ❖ By physicians verbal and non-verbal behavior [96].

A practice that came up in both nursing and physician communication, but more frequently related to physician communication, is that of nurses accompanying physicians on rounds, which promotes the proportionate messaging idea expressed in daily meetings. Many hospitals provide chairs or stools in patient rooms to encourage physicians to sit down during patient rounds and conduct a less rushed and more concerned feel to physician communication [92].

Important Strategies here;

- ❖ Data feedback, friendly competition
- ❖ Nurses accompany physicians on rounds
- ❖ Sit down during patient visits
- ❖ Note pads and pens at bedside for patient questions
- ❖ Engaged physician leaders
- ❖ Hospitalist programs [91].

Responsiveness of hospital staff

This essentially demonstrates how satisfied patients are with the amount of time it takes hospital staff to respond to requests for help. Hourly rounding is by far the most common procedure presented as an important driver of patient satisfaction related to hospital staff responsiveness in both lower and higher volume critical access hospitals [91,92].

Hourly Rounding

Hourly rounding refers to meaningful patient visits managed by licensed or unlicensed nursing staff to check on the patient's condition and take care of personal needs, essentially, before the patient has to push a call light. Almost 65 percent of the participating critical access hospitals attribute hourly rounding to patient satisfaction related to responsiveness of hospital staff. Several participants add that hourly rounding ultimately contributes to staff satisfaction as well due to a subsequent decrease in patient call light use by patients. Hourly rounds are often structured around what is commonly known as the "4 P's – pain, potty, position, and personal effects or possessions", and usually end with staff asking patients "Is there anything I can get you before I go?" [91].

No Pass Zone

It is a concept that everyone wearing a hospital badge is responsible to answer call lights or patient alarms, often referred to as the "no pass zone." Patient care requests for non-clinical support such as a beverage or tissue are taken care of immediately by any employee, including the CEO, while requests of a clinical nature are handed off to nursing personnel. Overall, comments related to no pass zone are positive with an added quipped perk of less traffic in patient care areas due to avoidance by staff afraid to enter patient rooms [91].

Technological Devices

Technological devices thought to improve response times by hospital staff involve call light system characteristics and nursing communication devices, some of which were connected. Bed alarms can be integrated into call light systems, flashing different colors outside the room and sounding different alarms. Nursing communication devices ranged from old school pagers to handheld phones integrated with the call light system to hands-free ear pieces that allow nurses to communication with patients and with other nurses on different channels [91].

Pain Management

Patients are given an opportunity to evaluate how well hospitals do in managing their pain on HCAHPS surveys. Several of the participants admitted that pain management is a difficult topic due to opioid abuse, but the overall atmosphere of the discussions were positive and proactive. Nurses are taught to use the words 'Let's see if this will help your pain [92,97].

The most frequent pain management interventions described by focus group participants are the use of patient whiteboards to document pain related information, discussing expectations and goals with patients, alternative therapies, and automated pain re-assessment reminders [91].

Alternative pain therapies are more frequently related as drivers of pain satisfaction regarding pain in lower volume critical access hospital focus groups. Therapies suggested include those involving heat or cold such as warm compresses, towels, blankets, and ice packs, as well as positioning, relaxing music, aroma therapy, distraction activities, pet therapy and back rubs or massage [91].

Communication about Medications

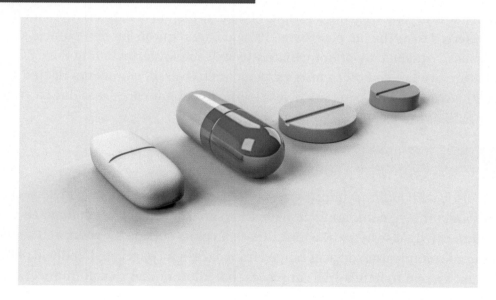

Focus group participants most commonly attribute success in this dimension to patient education provided by a pharmacist, closely followed by variations of written patient education on medications. Discharge phone calls, in some hospitals conducted by a pharmacist, medication reconciliation, and using key words such as "education on your medications" and "side effects of your medications" are other practices that are thought to drive HCAHPS communication about medication scores.

On pharmacist visits, it's recommended for the pharmacist to visit and inform patients about medications and side effects. Nurses used to do this, but the fresh face has helped scores immensely. Another helpful practice identified is for nurses to specify in simple terms what medications are for every time they are given, such as "for your heart" or "for your stomach" [91,92].

Cleanliness of Hospital Environment

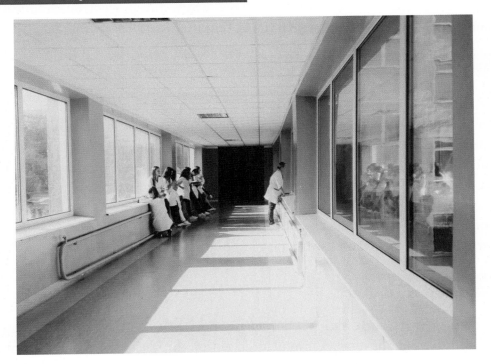

All staff members are responsible to scan a patients room and make sure things are picked up and the garbage is empty before they leave.

Key Strategies;

- ➢ Cleanliness auditing
- ➢ Notices of cleaning services
- ➢ Cleaning schedules
- ➢ Everyone is responsible for cleanliness
- ➢ Environmental services staff engagement as an integral part of the health care team
- ➢ Environmental services staff education on cleaning
- ➢ Environmental services staff education on customer service
- ➢ Access to environmental services staff via two-way radios or electronic requests
- ➢ Patient and Family Advisory Council (PFAC) environmental assessments [91].

Quietness of Hospital Environment

The need for rest in order to heal is a paradoxical idea given the bustling activity found in most hospitals. The HCAHPS question on quietness of the hospital environment challenges hospital leaders to find solutions to relieve that paradoxical tension. Heightened awareness through ongoing and frequent reminders was most regularly cited as a strategy. Staff reminders are provided in meetings, newsletters, e-mails, and in real time when voices are carrying or groups of people are congregating in hallways near patient rooms. Technological devices utilized to monitor and draw staff attention to noise levels have been used, and most participants agreed that the usefulness of these devices is, at best, short term to heighten awareness to noise levels [91].

Discharge Information

Generally, hospitals receive fairly high patient ratings on the HCAHPS topic of discharge information. For discharge information, the most common interventions are categorized broadly into three areas – discharge planning, discharge education, and discharge follow up, summarized in order of flow rather than by number of responses.

Discharge Planning

Discharge planning may be led by a social worker, discharge planning nurse, case manager, or a combination of all three, often in conjunction with a charge nurse and physician. The discharge planning leader begins rounding with patients early in their stay, in some hospitals accompanied by an interdisciplinary team. Planning begins with a baseline assessment of home needs and services, with the general goal of making sure patient needs will be met when they are discharged [91].

Discharge Phone Calls or Home Visits

Post discharge follow up, whether by phone or in person, is the most frequently referenced strategy connected to HCAHPS discharge information success. Strategies for implementation vary widely. Discharge phone calls might be conducted by a utilization review nurse, discharge coordinator or planner, or pharmacist, most often two to three days after discharge. Patients are asked about their pain, if they have questions about their medications, and discharge information might be reviewed. Some hospitals follow up only with certain types of patients, such as obstetric or surgical patients or those deemed to be at a high risk of readmission. Several of the hospitals provide follow up home visits, most often based on criteria such as qualifying for home or community-based social services, high risk of readmission, or lack of access to home care services [91].

Care Transitions Strategies

- ❖ Community care collaboration
- ❖ Readmission committee
- ❖ Care transition programs
- ❖ Giving patients control of their care
- ❖ Explaining patient responsibilities
- ❖ "We want to have a good understanding of your references related to discharge needs"
- ❖ Staff education on the HCAHPS survey questions [90,92].

Patient-centered care organizational status checklist

Sampled patients are surveyed between 48 hours and six weeks after discharge, regardless of the mode of survey administration. Interviewing or distributing surveys to patients while they are still in the hospital is not permitted. Check your organizational readiness for improving patient care experience [90,92];

1. Are you collecting patient care experience data? Yes No (go to Q8)
2. How are you collecting patient care experience data?
3. Why are you collecting patient care experience data?
4. How often are you collecting patient care experience data?
5. How are you using the data/information collected?
6. Is the data about patient care experience being reported?
7. To whom is it being reported?
8. Is staff satisfaction monitored?
9. Is there a 'dashboard' of performance metrics monitored by the organization?
10. Does the 'dashboard'/set of metrics include patient care experience indicators?
11. What is the mission/vision of the organization?
12. What is the main message to staff from the leadership? CEO? Organizational governance?
13. Is the culture of the organization supportive of change? Open to learning?
14. Are successes by staff visibly celebrated?
15. What is the current area of focus for staff development?
16. Have staff training activities included communication skills training or patient-centered values?
17. Are patients and families considered 'partners' in care?
18. Are any patient or family/carer representatives involved in any organizational committees?
19. If so, which areas do these committees cover?
20. Any future plans for engaging patients at a service level within the organization?
21. Have there been any tragic events within the service from which lessons have been learnt? What did the organization learn from these events?
22. Are families/caregivers considered 'visitors' to the service (ie restricted 'visiting' hours)?

What must hospitals do in order to participate in HCAHPS?

CMS has developed detailed Rules of Participation and Minimum Survey Requirements for hospitals that either self-administer the survey or administer the survey for multiple hospital sites, and for survey vendors that conduct HCAHPS for client hospitals. The HCAHPS Rules of Participation include the following activities:

- ❖ Attend HCAHPS Introduction and Update Training
- ❖ Follow the Quality Assurance Guidelines and Policy Updates
- ❖ Certification of the accuracy of the organization's data collection process
- ❖ Develop a HCAHPS Quality Assurance Plan
- ❖ Become a QualityNet Exchange Registered User for data submission
- ❖ Participate in oversight activities conducted by the HCAHPS Project Team.

Hospitals and survey vendors administering the survey must also meet HCAHPS Minimum Survey Requirements with respect to survey experience, survey capacity, and quality control procedures. Details about these activities and requirements can be found in the Quality Assurance Guidelines under "Quality Assurance" at www.hcahpsonline.org [90-95].

Which patients are eligible to participate in HCAHPS?

The HCAHPS survey is widely proposed for patients of all payer types that meet the following criteria:

- ❖ 18 years or older at the time of presentation
- ❖ At least one overnight stay in the hospital as an inpatient
- ❖ Non-psychiatric diagnosis at discharge
- ❖ Alive at the time of discharge

Patients who meet these criteria (except those that fall into an exclusion category, described below) should be included in the sample frame from which the survey sample is drawn [90-95].

There are a few categories of otherwise eligible patients who, because of logistical difficulties in collecting data, are excluded from the sample frame before the random sample is selected. These are:

- ❖ Patients discharged to hospice care
- ❖ Patients discharged to nursing homes and skilled nursing facilities
- ❖ Court/Law enforcement patients (i.e., prisoners)
- ❖ Patients with a foreign home address (excluding U.S. territories—Virgin Islands, Puerto Rico, and Northern Mariana Islands)
- ❖ "No-Publicity" patients
- ❖ Patients who are excluded because of rules or regulations of the state in which the hospital is located [90-95].

V

Satisfaction and patients with spine diseases

Patient Selection for Spine Surgery

Unlike other musculoskeletal disorders, the etiology of back pain is often difficult to resolve and needs clear indications and criteria for surgical or nonsurgical intervention.

Correlating imaging findings with pain is unreliable most of times, and poor results are clearly associated with inaccurate patient selection or not proper treatment.

A careful history and physical examination, as well as a trial of non-operative management when convenient, are vital to the process of deciding whether or not a patient might benefit from surgical intervention.

The most challenging patients are those who suffer back pain with no neurologic deficit, no radicular pain, no instability, no deformity, and who have not responded to a strict medical management program.

Patients with low back pain should be worked up on a case-by-case basis. Provocative testing can be used as an accessory to diagnostic imaging in selected cases.

A correct relevant extensive preoperative evaluation of the patient status is mandatory.

The pathology had a lot to do with patient satisfaction.

Several parameters have also impact on satisfaction even if not related to the pathology like depression, employment, insurance and so on.

What patients expect from spine surgery is important as it relates to patient satisfaction [98].

Even if the clinical expectations were met, some patients will be dissatisfied.

Patients with spinal stenosis seems to have more overestimated expectation, same with deformity.

The surgeon experience and capability and theatre facilities plays integral rule in achieving satisfaction.

Choose the right patient for spinal surgery.

Patient expectations

Preoperative patient expectations about the surgical results are a significantly vital cause of patient satisfaction with spinal surgery. Preoperative expectations in spine surgery refers to patient preferences with relation to postoperative outcome linked to patient symptomatology or function. Patient satisfaction refers to patient's belief related to a specific symptom or function, which may be unyielding as current satisfaction at follow-up or as percent achievement of preoperatively established expectations. Previous surveys have showed lower postoperative satisfaction in patients with incoherent expectations before undergoing total joint replacement and spinal decompression. Other studies have revealed that patients with higher expectation of success in spine surgery report better satisfaction. There is also some evidence to promote that preoperative expectations play a role in the postoperative functional outcome. However, there is no general acceptance, and it remains unrecognized whether preoperative expectations in lumbar surgery affect the postoperative satisfaction or functional outcomes.

One of the primary objectives patients seek lumbar spine surgery is for alleviation of pain. Sadly, due to the indolent nature of spine surgery, including etiology, chronicity of symptoms, and medical and surgical history, it is difficult to predict which patients will experience the greatest symptom relief. As surgeons counsel their patients, it is vital to understand the significance of patient expectations for pain on satisfaction and outcome. Although the results presented everywhere are mixed, demonstrating a fascinating interaction for leg pain and back pain, it is vital to keep in mind the multimodal donations to patient pain [98,99,100].

In a study done by Saniya S. Godil et al [101], on 500 patients undergoing elective spine surgery for degenerative conditions over a 6-month time at a single medical center were included into a prospective longitudinal study. Data collected on all patients included demographics, disease characteristics, treatment variables, readmissions/reoperations, and all 90-day surgical morbidity. Patient-reported outcome instruments (NRS, ODI, NDI, SF-12, EQ-5D, Zung depression scale, and MSPQ anxiety scale), return to work, patient satisfaction with outcome, and patient satisfaction with provider care were recorded at baseline and 3 months after treatment. Multifaceted logistic regression analysis was practiced to certify if surgical morbidity (quality) or bettering in disability and quality of life (effectiveness of care) were independently associated with patient satisfaction. They conclude that patient satisfaction is not a valid measure of overall quality or effectiveness of surgical spine care. Patient satisfaction metrics likely represent the patient's subjective fulfillment with health-care service, a separate aspect of care. Satisfaction measures are important patient-centered scope of health-care service but should not be used as a score for overall quality, safety, or effectiveness of surgical spine care.

In spite of that, **even if the clinical expectation were met, some patients were still dissatisfied**. Patients with spinal stenosis seem to have more unrealistic expectations than patients with disc prolapse [102].

In the study of a total of 1645 patients underwent elective spine surgery, for degenerative lumbar and cervical disease over a period of 2 years were enrolled in a prospective longitudinal registry, done by Silky Chotai et al [103]. Patient-reported outcome, the Oswestry Disability Index (ODI)/Neck Disability Index (NDI), and numeric rating scale for back pain/neck pain (BP/NP) and leg/arm pain (LP/AP), were recorded at baseline and the 12-month follow-up. Patient satisfaction was evaluated with the North American Spine Society Satisfaction Questionnaire. They found that uninsured payer status and higher baseline pain scores were the independent predictors of patient dissatisfaction at 12 months after surgery.

An analysis of prospectively collected multicenter data, done by Alexandra Soroceanu et al [104], to assess the link between preoperative expectations and postoperative outcomes and satisfaction in lumbar and cervical spine surgery.

In this study, the greater achievement of expectations led to higher postoperative satisfaction and was associated with better functional outcomes. Higher preoperative expectations led to decreased postsurgical satisfaction but were associated with improved functional outcomes. Higher postoperative satisfaction was associated with improved functional outcomes and vice versa. Type of surgery also affected satisfaction and function, with cervical patients being less satisfied but having better functional outcomes than lumbar patients. This study showed that more than functional outcomes matter; preoperative expectations and achievement of expectations affect postoperative satisfaction in patients undergoing lumbar and cervical spine surgery. This emphasizes the importance of taking preoperative expectations in consideration to obtain an informed choice on the basis of the patient's preferences.

Microendoscopic Diskectomy

Conventional techniques (open diskectomy and microdiskectomy) are considered the gold standard techniques that spinal surgeons used to decompress symptomatic lumbar nerve roots effectively. There has been increasing interest in using an endoscopic, minimally invasive surgical approach.

Since Foley and Smith described the Microendoscopic diskectomy MED technique in 1997 for radicular decompression in patients with lumbar herniated disk, good initial results with little complications, even in cases with a component of associated stenosis, have been published more and more frequently [105].

Patient satisfaction with surgery was good in 95% of the patients at the final review. In a longitudinal, prospective study done by Roberto Casal-Moro et al [106], the study was based on 120 patients with a diagnosis of herniated lumbar disk who were treated with MED. The results were assessed with the VAS pain score, Oswestry Disability Index score, patient satisfaction questionnaire, and modified Macnab criteria. The results at the final review (5) years were good or excellent in 75% of patients and regular in 18%. Good subjective satisfaction was noticed with surgery in 92% of patients.

Fair results in 18.3%, and poor results in 7.5%. In summary, 75.8% of the patients returned to their usual job activity (mean time, 8.1weeks), 13.3% had to perform another activity, and 6.7% were assigned incapacity benefit.

Smoking

Tobacco use has been related to pathophysiology of poor tissue healing and lower fusion rates after lumbar spine surgery (toxic to osteoblast). Retrospective studies have suggested that smoking status could be an important negative predictor of outcomes, equally as important as preoperative severity and duration of symptoms. Historically, smoking patients admitted for spinal disease have worse outcome, elevated complications, and more costs than nonsmokers.

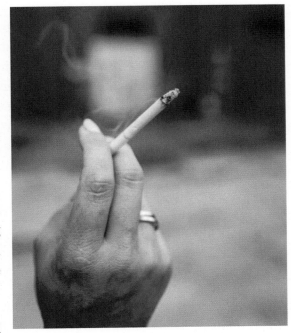

Smoking has been associated with worse self-reported outcomes and less improvement in patients sustaining lumbar spine surgery. Accordingly, smoking is identified as a significant risk factor for complications after spine surgery [107].

In one prospective study included 5100 patients operated for central spinal stenosis without degenerative spondylolisthesis, Sigmundsson and colloquies [108] found that 88 % of the patients sustained decompression only and 12 % had decompression and fusion. The aim of the study was to assess motivations of patient satisfaction 1 year after surgery for central spinal stenosis without degenerative spondylolisthesis. They found that there were serious baseline differences between satisfied and dissatisfied patients in all patient reported outcome measures except leg pain. Factors limiting the likelihood for satisfaction included;

❖ Previous spine surgery
❖ Smoking
❖ Unemployment

❖ Back pain exceeding 1 year
❖ Back pain predominance

Preoperative self-estimated walking distance more than 1000 meter predicted satisfaction, though fusion surgery did not predict satisfaction [108,109,110].

In a prospective cohort study, done by Laura Chapin, Kelly Ward and Timothy Ryken [111] on 166 patients who underwent lumbar spine surgeries at Iowa Spine and Brain Institute to assess whether comorbidities and demographics, recognized preoperatively, can affect patient outcomes and satisfaction after lumbar spine surgery. Preoperative smoking status, self-reported depression, prevalence of diabetes, obesity, level of education, and employment status were estimated in the context of patient outcome and satisfaction after lumbar spine surgery. Patients were assessed before surgery, and at 3 and 12 months postoperatively, and responded to Oswestry Disability Index (ODI) and EuroQol-5 Dimensions (EQ-5D) self-assessment examinations, as well as a satisfaction measure. Depression, smoking, and employment status were found to be significant elements in patient satisfaction. Depressed patients, smokers, and patients on disability at the time of surgery have worse ODI and EQ-5D scores at all of the time points (baseline, 3 months, and 12 months post-surgery).

Preoperative diagnosis

In a study done by Charles H. Crawford III and colloquies [112] to determine if the preoperative diagnosis—disc herniation, stenosis, spondylolisthesis, adjacent segment degeneration, or mechanical disc collapse—would affect patient satisfaction after surgery. Patients enrolled in the Quality Outcomes Database, formerly known as the National Neurosurgery Quality and Outcomes Database (N2QOD), completed patient-reported outcome measures, including the Oswestry Disability Index (ODI) and Numeric Rating Scale (NRS) for back pain (NRS-BP) and leg pain (NRS-LP) preoperatively and 1-year postoperatively. Patients were laminated by diagnosis and by their response to the satisfaction question:

❖ Surgery met my expectations
❖ I did not improve as much as I hoped, but I would undergo the same operation for the same results;
❖ Surgery helped, but I would not undergo the same operation for the same results; or
❖ I am the same or worse as compared with before surgery.

A greater percentage of patients with primary disc herniation or spondylolisthesis reported that surgery met expectations (66% and 67%, respectively), followed by recurrent disc herniation and stenosis (59% and 60%, respectively). A smaller percentage of patients who underwent surgery for adjacent segment degeneration or mechanical disc collapse had their expectations met (48% and 41%, respectively).

The proportion of patients that would undergo the same surgery again, by diagnostic category, was as follows: disc herniation 88%, recurrent disc herniation 79%, spondylolisthesis 86%, stenosis 82%, adjacent segment disease 75%, and mechanical collapse 73%. Whatever the diagnosis, mean improvement and ultimate 1-year postoperative ODI, NRS-BP, and NRS-LP reflected patient satisfaction. They conclude that the preoperative diagnosis was predictive of patient satisfaction following spine surgery.

Moreover, Alrawi et al [113], in a prospective case series concluded that preoperative neurophysiologic studies can help to define which patients are more likely to gain from surgery for cervical radiculopathy. This study provides Level III diagnostic evidence that patients with cervical radiculopathy and an MRI showing a disc bulge with narrowing of the exiting foramina have better clinical outcomes and patient satisfaction from ACDF if a preoperative EMG shows denervation changes.

Obesity

Health-related factors such as diabetes, obesity, and smoking considerably affect surgical outcomes and complications. Studies have resolved an increase in surgical site infections in morbidly obese patients [98].

[www.pixabay.com]

Obesity has been shown to be a considerable factor in the development of musculoskeletal disease. In particular, there has been a recent rising interest in the role of obesity in lumbar spine disease and surgical outcomes for lumbar spine pathology. Obese patients are more likely to develop both clinical and radiographic evidence of degenerative lumbar spine disease. Weight loss, whether in the form of diet and exercise regimens or bariatric surgery, may afford some improvement in clinical lumbar spine complaints. In cases in which surgery is necessary to treat degenerative lumbar spine pathology, obese patients experience improvement but less so compared to non-obese patient. Obese patients may be more chance to develop perioperative and postoperative complications [114].

The association between obesity and satisfaction following lumbar spinal surgery has been inconsistent. In a large-registry study based on the Swedish Spine Registry of 2633 lumbar stenosis patients, Knutsson and colloquies [115], found that obese patients, in general, had less satisfaction following surgery. A higher BMI was linked with greater odds of dissatisfaction and poorer outcomes after surgery for lumbar spinal stenosis and lower results at the 2-year follow-up. However, in a study by McGuire and colleagues [116], there was no difference between obese and non-obese patients in symptom satisfaction at 12 months following surgery particularly for degenerative lumbar spondylolisthesis. BMI was not a significant independent predictor of satisfaction. This suggests that other factors (for example, patient sex) may be more important for preoperative counseling and the assessment of which patients will be most satisfied after surgery for degenerative lumbar spondylolisthesis.

Another Population-based retrospective cohort study, done by Cinzia Gaudelli and Ken Thomas [117], to determine if the patients with a body mass index (BMI) ≥35 undergoing elective lumbar spine surgery are at higher risk of postoperative complications, as defined by reoperation within a 3-month period?, and also to assess if there are any patient subgroups at a higher risk of reoperation? Subgroups, included gender, age, location of surgery (urban versus rural setting), and type of procedure performed (decompression, decompression with instrumented fusion, deformity correction, and arthroplasty). They found that in obese patients increasing of complication rate after elective lumbar spine surgery, as evidenced by reoperation rates within 3 months. When they determined other possible associations with reoperation, in adjusted analysis, deformity surgery was found to be predictive of early reoperation.

Coronary artery disease

The association between coronary artery disease and lower outcomes following lumbar spinal surgery, in general, is clearer. In a systematic review done by Aalto TJ, and colloquies, of 21 studies on preoperative predictors of outcomes of surgery for lumbar spinal stenosis, cardiovascular comorbidity was associated with poor patient satisfaction at the 2-year follow-up.

Increased attention to cardiac comorbidities may be considered to optimize satisfaction following surgery for degenerative lumbar spondylolisthesis [118].

In a retrospective analysis of a prospective, national longitudinal registry don by Andrew K Chan et al [119], which including patients whom underwent surgery for grade 1 degenerative lumbar spondylolisthesis. The most and least satisfied patients were marked based on an answer of "1" and "4," respectively, on the North American Spine Society (NASS) Satisfaction Questionnaire 12 months postoperatively. Baseline demographics, clinical variables, surgical parameters, and outcomes were collected. Patient-reported outcome measures, including the Numeric Rating Scale (NRS) for back pain, NRS for leg pain, Oswestry Disability Index (ODI), and EQ-5D (the EuroQol health survey), were conducted at baseline and 3 and 12 months after treatment. In an analysis of 477 patients undergoing surgery they found that 255 patients (53.5%) determined as most satisfied and 26 (5.5%) determined as least satisfied 12 months after the index surgery. The most satisfied patients had a significantly lower mean BMI and a lower rate of CAD (coronary artery disease).

Gender

Female sex was independently associated with the most satisfaction at 12 months after surgery. While in prior investigations of lumbar spinal surgery, female sex was associated with inferior or equivocal satisfaction [120,121]

Psychological status

In a prospective-registry study done by Chapin L and colloquies [111] of 166 patients who had undergone lumbar spine surgery at a single center, they found that depression, smoking, and employment status were significant predictors of patient satisfaction. Other studies have shown worse satisfaction following lumbar spinal surgery in patients with depression and smoking [111,122].

In a study done by Robert K Merilli and colloquies [123] to investigate the effect depression has on the improvement of patient-reported outcome measures (PROMs) following lumbar decompression. They found that depressed patients have worse postoperative outcomes for patient-reported outcome measures PROMIS physical function, depression, pain, and ODI. These findings are important for risk assessment and treating depressed patients before lumbar spine decompression.

ASA class

The literature has also shown the ASA class to predict patient satisfaction following lumbar spine surgery. In a study by Mannion and colleagues [124], the percentage of patients satisfied with surgery was 87%, 85%, and 79% for preoperative ASA classes I, II, and III, respectively, indicating that higher ASA classes were associated with lower rate of patient satisfaction. In contrast to these studies, our study focused only on patients with lumbar spondylolisthesis; thus, the differing pathology-specific factors may have contributed to the differences reported herein.

Fusion surgery

Currently, there is a drive in the spine community to implement more prospective analyses, comparing treatment strategies along with outcome analyses using recognized scales, such as the Oswestry Low Back Pain Disability Questionnaire and the 36-Item Short Form Health Survey (SF-36).

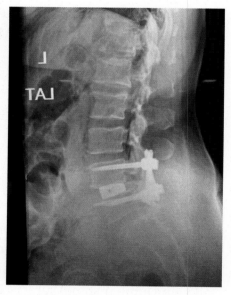

These analyses report patient satisfaction and quality of life after procedures, rather than fusion rate and neurologic recovery.

The former are the ultimate goals and the true motivations of treatment efficacy [125].

Circumferential lumbar fusion is a valid procedure for a patient with difficult reconstructive disease. There is a very high fusion rate (up to 99%) in one study. Overall, 62% of patients are satisfied with the outcome, especially those with a diagnosis of pseudarthrosis or spondylolisthesis with stenosis. Patients who are working before surgery and patients who are not injured workers also tended to progress well.

In a review done by Slosar and colloquies [126], of 141 consecutive patients who underwent instrumented circumferential lumbar fusions. Outcome was assessed by an independent third party. The clinical outcomes and the assessment of patient satisfaction done after a minimum follow-up of 2 years.

In this study, (11%) of the patients chose the statement, "surgery met my expectations"; (51%) chose, "surgery improved my condition enough that I would go through it again for the same outcome"; (20%)

chose, "surgery helped me but I would not go through it again for the same outcome"; and (19%) chose, "I am the same or worse compared with before surgery."

There was no statistical difference in patient satisfaction between primary and revision surgeries or between workers' compensation versus non-workers' compensation groups.

While Crawford, et al [112], report that greater proportion of patients in general undergoing surgery for spondylolisthesis reported high satisfaction postoperatively, as compared with those undergoing surgery for other lumbar pathologies, such as recurrent disc herniation, stenosis, adjacent segment degeneration, or mechanical disc collapse. Thus, surgery for degenerative lumbar spondylolisthesis remains an important treatment option in well-selected patients.

Scoliosis

Patients with progressive idiopathic scoliosis may have several evident body deformities, including scapular and rib prominence, uneven shoulders, and an asymmetric waistline. Spinal fusion surgery with instrumentation often successfully reduces severe curves and minimizes the risk of curve progression. Unluckily, success of surgical technique does not necessarily reflected into patient satisfaction.

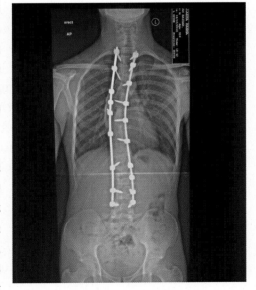

Patient satisfaction with spinal surgery has largely been assessed in retrospective studies and most consistently is related to postoperative cosmesis and percentage of curve correction. Most adolescents with idiopathic scoliosis expressed satisfaction with the cosmetic surgical result. Preoperative physical components, psychological difficulties, and overestimated expectations regarding postoperative cosmesis are correlated with patient dispassion or dissatisfaction [127,128].

The rate of correction was directly correlated with satisfaction. In other words, the greater correction reflects in more satisfaction and better quality of life. Cosmesis and appearance is the most vital factor affecting patient's satisfaction and quality of life. Although patients with AIS have no concern about pain and functional limitations, it seems that the most important obsession of these patients is the appearance which should be considered in treatment planning. Surgery was associated with improved patient's self-image, psychology, and satisfaction while pain and function remained unchanged [127,128].

In their study, Ameri and colloquies [129] found that total SRS score improved significantly after surgery.

Fifty per cent of patients revealed satisfaction with the postoperative appearance of their back after surgical correction of severe curve. Neutral or dissatisfied patients, with an otherwise satisfactory medical outcome, had identifiable differences in preoperative medical and psychological variables in comparison with their satisfied siblings. Patients who underwent anterior and posterior fusion generally expressed more disappointment with the postoperative appearance of their scar but expressed greater satisfaction with their back and shoulders than did the patients who underwent posterior fusion.

Neutral or dissatisfied patients, in general, were more likely to be thin and have King II or King IV curve types than were satisfied patients.

Likewise, dissatisfied female patients were also more likely to be younger in menarcheal age than their satisfied counterparts. Thus, the orthopedist should be particularly sensitive to thin girls who are premenarchal or have a younger menarchal status, because they may be strictly susceptible to dissatisfaction with the cosmetic outcome. Neutral or dissatisfied patients were more likely to report a history of sadness, anxiety, loneliness, problems with relationships, and negative self-perception before surgery than satisfied patients.

Patient age

Patient satisfaction is multimodal and not only concomitant with improvement in the calculated outcome parameters. Patient expectations, preoperative health issues and psychological distress may impact satisfaction after surgery.

Elderly obese patients undergoing lumbar surgery report a high rate of dissatisfaction with the surgery outcome compared with non-obese patients [98].

Generally, elderly patients have more comorbidities. As the number of preoperative comorbidities increase, more complications develop.

In the review study of Jin-Young Lee and colloquies [130], they found there was no increasing tendency of complications after spinal surgery in geriatric patients in one nonrandomized prospective, three case-control and four case series studies. However, postoperative complications increased in three case series studies, especially in patients over 80 years old. Luckily, most postoperative complications after spine surgery in elderly patients were minor.

The clinical outcome after spine surgery was satisfactory in geriatric patients with age between 65 and 101 after 2 to 8 years of follow-up period. Addition of arthrodesis had no adverse effect on the clinical outcomes.

Glassman, et al. [131,132] investigated clinical outcomes of 224 patients following lumbar decompression and arthrodesis for spinal stenosis. Patients were divided into two groups according to ages; over (n=50) or below 65 years old (n=174). The health related quality-of-life measures (HRQOL) including Oswestry Disability Index (ODI), the Medical Outcomes Study Short Form-36 (SF-36), back pain VAS, and leg pain VAS were evaluated for the mean follow-up of two years. There was no difference in the postoperative clinical outcomes. They conducted another study on postoperative clinical outcomes of 178 patients following lumbar decompression and arthrodesis for spinal stenosis or spondylolisthesis. Patients were divided into two groups according to ages; over (n=85) or below 65 years old (n=93). There was no difference in the clinical outcomes with the mean follow-up of 33 months, evaluated with the same HRQOL.

In conclusion, there was no difference in clinical outcome, postoperative complication and mortality rates between geriatric and non-geriatric patients. However, there is insufficient evidence to make strong recommendations with regard to spinal surgery for geriatric patients with lumbar stenosis and spondylolisthesis. High-quality, prospective randomized studies on the spinal surgery for geriatric patients with lumbar stenosis and spondylolisthesis are needed.

Cervical laminoplasty is a considerably accepted treatment for patients with cervical spondylotic myelopathy, and many reports have proved satisfactory outcomes. However, surgical outcomes of laminoplasty in elderly patients with cervical spondylotic myelopathy are controversial. Many reports have indicated lower surgical outcomes in elderly patients, while other reports have described no significant differences in surgical outcomes between elderly and non-elderly patients [133]. In a systematic review and meta-analysis conducted by Yasuhiro Takeshima and colloquies [134] to determine differences in surgical outcomes of laminoplasty for cervical spondylotic myelopathy between elderly and non-elderly patients. Nine clinical studies that met all inclusion criteria were included in the meta-analysis. A total of 1817 patients in these studies underwent cervical laminoplasty. They found that the elderly patients had lower preoperative and postoperative Japanese Orthopedic Association (JOA) scores, and lower recovery rates based on JOA scores. They also found that there are poor surgical outcomes and lower preoperative JOA scores in elderly patients. So they recommend that early surgical intervention may be suggested in elderly patients with cervical spine myelopathy CSM.

Another study done by Nan Su, et al, [135] found also that the age, preoperative JOA scores, and preoperative image signal intensity were the independent factors that significantly affect disease prognosis and surgical outcomes.

In 2007, the Japanese Orthopaedic Association Cervical Myelopathy Evaluation Questionnaire (JOACMEQ) was developed to compensate the conventional JOA score. This new self-administered questionnaire consists of 24 questions and includes patients' satisfaction, disability, handicaps, and general health. An English version is available.

Factors that can anticipate the outcome of laminoplasty include the patient's age, period of disease, severity of disease, preoperative cervical kyphosis, transverse area of the spinal cord, occupying ratio of the OPLL, and preoperative signal changes on magnetic resonance imaging (MRI) [136,137].

In an outcome study of PLIF of elderly patients (≥ 70 years of age), although no clear differences in the clinical results were observed, collapsed and delayed unions were more common and postoperative adjacent level disease was less frequent in the elderly patients, compared with younger patients (< 70 years of age) [138].

Another prospective cohort study done by Atsushi Kimura and colloquies, [139] to assess the predictors of patient satisfaction with outcome after cervical laminoplasty for compressive cervical myelopathy. They found that lower baseline QOL (quality of life) measured by SF-36 scores, specifically in bodily pain, general health perception, and vitality domains, are correlated to lower satisfaction with outcome after cervical laminoplasty.

In a study done by Jin-Young Lee and colloquies [130] to review the clinical outcome of spinal surgery in elderly patients with spinal stenosis or spondylolisthesis which are most commonly experienced in clinical practice of spinal surgeon. They found that the clinical outcome after spine surgery was satisfactory in geriatric patients with age between 65 and 101 after 2 to 8 years of follow-up period. Addition of arthrodesis had no adverse effect on the clinical outcomes.

In the complications, they found no increasing tendency after spinal surgery in geriatric patients in one nonrandomized prospective, three case-control and four case series studies. Nevertheless, postoperative complications increased in three case series studies, particularly in patients over 80 years old. Fortunately, most postoperative complications after spine surgery in elderly patients were minor [130].

Open and MIS

Muscle-sparing technology and approaches have been applied to spine surgery, decompression and fusion. The merits in short-term outcomes with muscle sparing are superior for pain, time to ambulation, hospital length of stay, and medication usage [140].

The application of MIS approaches to treat degenerative spine disease, including spondylolisthesis, is continuously rising among spinal surgeons. While there are many potential merits to the MIS approach, like shorter recovery time, reduced blood loss, and minimized soft-tissue damage with resultant reduction in postoperative pain and disability. There is still a gap of strong Class I evidence proving its efficacy and safety over conventional open approaches for the management of spondylolisthesis [141].

In a study done by Mummaneni et al [142], on 345 patients whom undergoing posterior lumbar fusion between July 2014 and December 2015 for Grade I degenerative spondylolisthesis. (open surgery, n = 254; MIS, n = 91) from 11 institutions across the United States. The authors recorded baseline and 12-month patient-reported outcomes (PROs), including Oswestry Disability Index (ODI), EQ-5D, numeric rating scale (NRS)–back pain (NRS-BP), NRS–leg pain (NRS-LP), and satisfaction (North American Spine Society satisfaction questionnaire). Multivariable regression models were fitted for hospital length of stay (LOS), 12-month PROs, and 90-day return to work, after modifying for a collection of preoperative and surgical variables. They found that both approaches are very effective in treating the underlying pathology and comforting back and leg pain and function. Overall, postoperative functional and surgical outcomes were equivalent between the MIS and open surgery subgroups. Moreover, patient satisfaction about the procedure and the postoperative recovery between the two groups were not statistically significant. Lastly, the rates for observed readmission and return to the operating room were very low in both groups.

Another published systematic review and meta-analysis of 10 studies including 602 patients reported that there was no significant difference in terms of functional or pain outcomes (ODI and visual analog scale, respectively), between open surgery and MIS [143].

A previous study done by Parker and colleagues [144] investigated 100 patients (50 in each arm) who underwent transforaminal interbody fusion (TLIF) for spondylolisthesis. The authors found similar surgical morbidity and hospital readmission rates for MIS and open TLIF.

In thoracolumbar trauma fracture, a study done by Barbagallo and colloquies [145] to assess the comparative effectiveness and safety of percutaneous minimally invasive versus open spine surgery for fractures of the thoracolumbar junction. They found that percutaneous MIS resulted in less blood loss and shorter length of hospital stay than open surgery. While radiographic outcomes were identical between treatment groups, and the patient function was statistically not significant between the two groups.

Motion preserving surgery

Discectomies, foraminotomies, and laminectomies are "tried and true" motion-preserving, non-implant operations with high rates of success when applied to the specific patient population. These decompressive operations should be actively considered as a prudent treatment options in patients with nerve root compression in the absence of spinal instability, spondylolisthesis, or deformity. It provides less chance of future adjacent-segment disease compared with laminectomy and fusion. It also avoids the costs and risks of implant insertion [146].

Motion preserving surgery has been developed in an attempt to limit the likelihood of intervertebral disc degeneration at segments adjacent to a fusion.

Classically, simple decompression surgery was motion preserving. More specific devices have been developed since.

The functional spinal unit (FSU) is defined as the smallest motion segment of the spine that express biomechanical characteristics representative of the physiologic motion of the entire spine. As the disc degenerates, a sequel of events ensues that eventually may result in symptomatic degenerative disc disease.

A dysfunctional motion segment is defined as an FSU that, for one reason or another, can no longer bear and resist the loads placed on it during daily activity without demonstrating abnormal motion and often pain.

By removing the dysfunctional joints and replacing them with a bony fusion, the abnormal motion of the motion segment is no longer present and the loads that were previously borne by that segment are now combined with the adjacent intact segments. This, many believe, is the driving force behind adjacent segment degeneration.

The ideal motion-sparing implant depicts the anatomy, motion, and mechanics of the intact, healthy FSU [147].

In a level one evidence, Prospective, multicenter, randomized clinical trial, Frank M. Phillips and colloquies [148-150], try to evaluate the long-term safety and effectiveness of the PCM (mobile) Cervical Disc compared with anterior cervical discectomy and fusion (ACDF) in treatment of patients with symptomatic single level degenerative spondylosis in subaxial cervical spine with or without prior cervical fusion. A total of 416 patients were randomized (224 PCM, 192 ACDF) at 24 investigational sites within the United States. Evaluations included patient-reported self-assessments, physical and neurological examination, and quantitative and qualitative radiographical analysis. Validated self-assessment outcomes measures included neck disability index (NDI) (a measure of pain-related dysfunction), 36-Item Short Form Health Survey (SF-36) mental and physical general health surveys (mental component summary and physical component summary), and neck and arm pain scores on a 0- to 100-mm visual analogue scale (VAS). At 5 years, the mean patient satisfaction VAS scores were 86.9/100 mm and 78.3/100 mm for the PCM and ACDF groups, respectively. Moreover the PCM group revealed greater improvements in neck pain, NDI, and general health, and higher patient satisfaction than the ACDF cohort. Rates of adverse events and secondary surgical procedures trended lower in the PCM cohort out to current follow-up of 7 years. Radiographical metrics revealed stability of PCM treatment over time, with continued motion (flexion/extension range of motion at the index level averaged 5.2 °, and no significant increase in heterotopic ossification or loss of disc height since 2-year results. Cervical arthroplasty is thought to protect adjacent levels; at 5 years, signs of adjacent-level degeneration were identified in statistically fewer levels adjacent to PCM than to ACDF [148-150].

On the other hand, Murrey et al, [151,152] conducted a prospective randomized controlled trial comparing safety and efficacy of TDA to ACDF for single level symptomatic cervical disc disease with radiculopathy. Of the 209 patients included in the study, 106 were assigned to the ACDF group and 103 to TDA. There was no difference in demographics between the TDA and ACDF groups. Follow-up rates were 98% for TDA and 94% for ACDF. ACDF had statistically significantly lower smaller blood loss and operative time (although differences small). Neurological improvement was better for TDA than ACDF at six months, but no significant difference was observed at 24 months. NDI improved from baseline for each group; however, between groups there was a significant difference at three months for TDA but not at 24 months. This was also true for aggregate patients who had greater than a 15 point improvement. Secondary surgical procedures were achieved in 1.9% of TDA patients and 8.5% of ACDF patients. Implant revision was needed in 4.7% of the ACDF patients, with 2.8% of the ACDF patients mandating supplemental fixation, while no TDA patients required revision. VAS neck pain, arm pain frequency and intensity were identical for TDA and ACDF patients at 24 months. Success, as defined by greater than 20% improvement in VAS scores, was expressed for 87.9% of TDA patients and 86.9% of ACDF patients at 24 months. At 24 months, 80.8% of TDA patients and 74.4% of ACDF patients had successful outcomes as assessed by the SF-36 physical component summary. The SF-36 mental component summary showed 71.8% of TDA and 68.9% of ACDF patients were successful. Patient satisfaction, narcotic use and adverse events were comparable for both groups. The authors concluded that TDA for single level disease is safe and effective and at least as good as ACDF.

Spinal stenosis

Park et al, [153] presented a retrospective comparative study looking at the SPORT study results to assess the impact of multilevel stenosis on surgical and medical/interventional treatment outcomes. Patients with three or more levels of stenosis had moderately less severe pain at baseline on the SF-36 bodily pain scale compared to one and two levels. Patients with single level stenosis were less likely to present with neurogenic claudication and more likely to report radicular pain radiation. Other baseline symptoms were similar in both groups. When comparing surgical to medical/interventional treatments for one, two and three level isolated stenosis, there was a significant surgical treatment impact in most outcomes measures within each subgroup at each time point. The only significant difference in treatment effects between subgroups was at two years for patient satisfaction with symptoms. Patients with single level stenosis had a lower difference in satisfaction between surgery and medical/interventional treatment, that is, a little treatment impact than the other two groups. This study provides Level III therapeutic evidence that patients with spinal stenosis without associated degenerative spondylolisthesis or scoliosis can be managed non-operatively irrelevant to the number of levels affected. If surgery is performed, the number of levels treated does not predict outcome [153].

Amundsen et al [154,155] performed a case control, comparative study of 100 patients with symptomatic spinal stenosis. Inclusion criteria were sciatic pain in the leg(s) with or without back pain and radiographic evidence of stenosis. These patients were separated into three groups: 19 patients with severe symptoms received surgical treatment, 50 patients with moderate symptoms received medical/ interventional management and 31 with moderate to severe symptoms were randomly assigned. The surgical group received decompression without fusion, inpatient rehabilitation with a brace, back school and physical therapy when out of the brace. The medical /interventional group was admitted to inpatient rehabilitation for one month, braced for up to three months, back school and physical therapy when out of brace. Patients were seen at regular intervals for 10 years. Authors assessed patients based on pain (no or light pain, moderate pain, severe pain), degree of stenosis and response to treatment (worse, unchanged, fair, excellent). With medical/interventional treatment, a good result was reported by 70% (35 of 50) of patients at six months, 64% (32 of 50) at one year and 57% (28 of 49) at four years. With surgery, a good result was reported by 79% (15 of 19) at six months, 89% (17 of 19) at one year and 84% (16 of 19) at four years. Of the patients randomly assigned to the medical/interventional group, good results were reported for 39% (seven of 18) at six months, 33% (six of 18) at one year and 47% (8 of 17) at four years. Of these patients, 56 % (10 of 18) reported being worse at six months.

Of the patients randomly enrolled to the surgical group, good results were reported for 92% (12 of 13) at six months, 69% (nine of 13) at one year and 92% (11 of 12) at four years. At the conclusion of 10 years, 10 patients in the medical/interventional group had died, 19 patients crossed over to surgery and 39 patients remained in this group. Of the patients remaining in the medical/interventional group, 70% experienced good results based on the assessment of pain.

In critique, no standardized outcome measures were utilized, and there were significant numbers of patient deaths and patients crossing over from medical/interventional to surgical treatment. Further, medical/interventional treatment consisted initially of a one-month stay on an inpatient rehabilitation unit for "back school" which is unlikely to apply in today's medical cost environment. In the randomized group, there is no direct statistical analysis comparing the surgical to the medical/interventional group. It is unclear that the results of initial treatment rendered differed from the natural history of spinal stenosis. Also, the medical/interventional group received minimal care (no injections, no indication of continued exercise program, etc).

The surgically treated group improved more than the medically/ interventionally treated group, although of the group with medical/interventional treatment, a large number of patients did quite well. This study provides Level II therapeutic evidence that patients with moderate to severe symptoms at presentation will receive a good result about 90% of the time compared with medical/interventional patients who will receive a good result only about 40% of the time. This study also supplies a level IV evidence that a cohort of patients with severe symptoms at presentation will have a good outcome with decompression 80-90% of the time and a cohort of patients with moderate symptoms will have a good result with medical/interventional treatment about 70% of the time [154,155].

Arinzon et al, [156,157] performed a prognostic case control study assessing the effect of decompression for lumbar spinal stenosis in elderly diabetic patients. The study included 62 diabetic patients and 62 gender- and age-matched non-diabetic controls. The mean follow-up was 40.3 months. Comorbidities were assessed and outcomes were measured using the visual analog scale (VAS), basic activities of daily living (BADL) and walking distance. The authors concluded that decompression for symptomatic spinal stenosis is valuable in elderly diabetic patients. However, the results are strongly affected by successful pain reduction, physical and mental health status, severity of clinical presentation, insulin treatment and duration of diabetes. The merits in diabetic patients are low as compared with non-diabetic patients with regard to symptom relief, satisfaction, BADL function and rate of complications.

In critique of this study, it highlights the clinical results of lumbar decompression in diabetic patients. Conclusions regarding mental health status were not supported with appropriate outcome tools to assess mental health. They failed to address the degree of stenosis in both the diabetic and control cohort. This study provides Level III prognostic evidence to support decompressive surgery for lumbar spinal stenosis in elderly diabetic patients. It also highlights the higher complication rate (p<0.0001) and less successful pain relief compared with non-diabetic patients (p=0.0067).

In the same line, Arinzon et al [157,158] conducted a previous retrospective, prognostic study of the effects of age on decompressive surgery for lumbar spinal stenosis. Two hundred eighty-three patients were divided according to age. One group was aged 65-74 years old and the second group was > 75-years-old. Follow-up was up to 42 months with a minimum of nine months. Within both treatment groups there was a significant (p<0.0001) subjective improvement in low back and radicular pain as well as the ability to perform daily activities. When compared to preoperative levels, the oral scores for pain while performing daily activities were significantly improved (p<0.001) in both treatment groups. The authors concluded that the overall postoperative complication rate was similar between the groups and that age is not a contraindication for surgical decompression of lumbar spinal stenosis. Both groups are equally likely to suffer minor perioperative complications. In critique of this study, there were no validated outcome tools and a lack of standardized surgical procedures, thus this paper provides Level III prognostic evidence that age greater than 75 years is not a contraindication for lumbar decompression compared with patients 65 to 74 years old.

References

1. https://dictionary.cambridge.org/dictionary/english/satisfaction

2. Param Hans Mishra, Tripti Mishra; Study of patient satisfaction at a super specialty tertiary care hospital. Indian Journal of Clinical Practice, Vol. 25, No. 7, December 2014.

3. Subashnie Devkaran; Patient experience is not patient satisfaction, understanding the fundamental differences. The International Society for Quality in healthcare. Webinar, November 2014.

4. Irwin Press, Patient satisfaction: understanding and managing the experience of care. 2nd ed., 2006 by the Foundation of the American College of Healthcare Executives. Health Administration Press.

5. Pamela L. Hudak, James G. Wright; The characteristics of patient satisfaction measures. SPINE Volume 25, Number 24, pp 3167–3177. 2000, Lippincott Williams & Wilkins, Inc.

6. Jackson JL, Chamberlin J, Kroenke K. Predictors of patient satisfaction. Soc Sci Med. 2001;52:609-20.

7. C Jenkinson, A Coulter, S Bruster, N Richards, T Chandola; Patients' experiences and satisfaction with health care: results of a questionnaire study of specific aspects of care. Qual Saf Health Care 2002;11:335–339.

8. Gavran, G.; "End-of-Life Choices a Vital Part of Patient Care." Health Leaders News, June 6, 2005. [Online article; retrieved 8/15/05.

9. http://www.healthleaders.com/news/print.php?contentid=68341

10. Jaipaul, C. K., and G. E. Rosenthal. "Do Hospitals with Lower Mortality Have Higher Patient Satisfaction?" American Journal of Medical Quality, 2003. 18 (2):59–65.

11. Peikes D, Chen A, Schore J, Brown R.; Effects of care coordination on hospitalization, quality of care, and health care expenditures among Medicare beneficiaries: 15 randomized trials. JAMA. 2009;301:603-18.

12. Manary MP, Boulding W, Staelin R, Glickman SW.; The patient experience and health outcomes. N Engl J Med. 2013;368:201-3.

13. Zolnierek KB, Dimatteo MR. Physician communication and patient adherence to treatment: a meta-analysis. Med Care. 2009;47:826-34.

14. Mitchell SE, Gardiner PM, Sadikova E, Martin JM, Jack BW, Hibbard JH, et al; Patient activation and 30-day post-discharge hospital utilization. J Gen Intern Med. 2014;29:349-55.

15. Kern LM, Dhopeshwarkar RV, Edwards A, Kaushal R.; Patient experience over time in patient-centered medical homes. Am J Manag Care. 2013; 19: 403-10.

16. Amgad N. Makaryus and Eli A. Friedman; Patients' understanding of their treatment plans and diagnosis at discharge. Mayo Clin Proc. August 2005;80(8):991-994.

17. Otani, K., Waterman, B., Faulkner, K. M., Boslaugh, S. & Claiborne, W. D.; How patient reactions to hospital care attributes affect the evaluation of overall quality of care, willingness to recommend, and willingness to return. Journal of Healthcare Management (2010), 55(1), 25-37.

18. Moerman, D. E. "Cultural Variation in the Placebo Effect: Ulcers, Anxiety, and Blood Pressure." Medical Anthropology Quarterly, 2000. 14 (1): 51–72.

19. Wolosin, R. J. "Patients' Perceptions of Safety in U.S. Hospitals." Poster presented at the Academy Health Annual Research Meeting, San Diego, 2004. CA, June 7-9.

20. Wolosin RJ, Vercler L, Matthews JL. Am I safe here?: improving patients' perceptions of safety in hospitals. J Nurs Care Qual. 2006 Jan-Mar;21(1):30-38; quiz 39-40.

21. Mayer, T., and R. Cates. Leadership for Great Customer Services: Satisfied Patients, Satisfied Employees. Chicago: Health Administration Press, 2004.

22. Lindsay E. Jubelt, et al; Patient ratings of case managers in a medical home: Associations with patient satisfaction and health care utilization. Ann Intern Med. 2014;161: S59-S65.

23. Renato Santos de Almeida, Stephane Bourliataux-Lajoinie, Mônica Martins; Satisfaction measurement instruments for healthcare service users: a systematic review. Cad. Saúde Pública, Rio de Janeiro, 31(1):11-25, jan, 2015.

24. Albert Yee, et al; Do patient expectations of spinal surgery relate to functional outcome?. Clin Orthop Relat Res (2008) 466:1154–1161.

25. Toyone T, Tanaka T, Kato D, Kaneyama R, Otsuka M.; Patients' expectations and satisfaction in lumbar spine surgery. Spine. 2005;30:2689–2694.

26. Katz JN, Stucki G, Lipson SJ, Fossel AH, Grobler LJ, Weinstein JN. Predictors of surgical outcome in degenerative lumbar spinal stenosis. Spine. 1999;24:2229–2233.

27. Eastaugh SR; Reducing litigation costs through better patient communication. Physician Exec. 2004 May-Jun;30(3):36-8.

28. David Lee Gordon; AIDET and the seven habits. Modified from original Studer Group presentation. https://www.studergroup.com/resources/healthcare-tools

29. Gregory Makoul, Amanda Zick, Marianne Green; An Evidence-Based Perspective on Greetings in Medical Encounters. Arch Intern Med. 2007;167(11):1172-1176.

30. Raul Zamora, Mitun Patel, Bryan Doherty, Adam Alperstein, Peter Devito; Influence of AIDET in the improving quality metrics in a small community hospital - before and after analysis. Journal of Hospital Administration. 2015, Vol. 4, No. 3. P 35-38.

31. Lynne Cunningham; Words Matter. MHS, Spring 2009. P 15-18.

32. Setia N, Meade C.; Bundling the value of discharge telephone calls and leader rounding. J Nurs Adm. 2009 Mar;39(3):138-41.

33. Kelley Moulds, Kenneth Epstein; Do post-discharge telephone calls to patients reduce the rate of complications? The Hospitalist. 2008 August; 2008(8).

34. Setia, N., & Meade, C.; Bundling the value of discharge telephone calls and leader rounding. Journal of Nursing Administration (2009), 39(3), 138-141.

35. Riegel B, Carlson B, Kopp Z, LePetri B, Glaser D, Unger A. Effect of a standardized nurse case-management telephone intervention on resource use in patients with chronic heart failure. Arch Intern Med. 2002 Mar 25;162(6):705-712.

36. Gardner, Glenn E., Woollett, Kaylene, Daly, Naomi, & Richardson, Bronwyn. Measuring the effect of patient comfort rounds on practice environment and patient satisfaction: a pilot study. International Journal of Nursing Practice (2009), 15(4), 287-293.

37. Halm, Margo A.; Hourly Rounds: What does the evidence indicate? American Journal of Critical Care (2009), 18(6), 581-584.

38. Christine M Meade, Amy L Bursell, and Lyn Ketelsen; Effects of nursing rounds: on patients' call light use, satisfaction, and safety. AJN The American Journal of Nursing. 106(9):58-70, September 2006.

39. Dempsey, C., Reilly, B., & Buhlman, N.; Improving the patient experience: Real-world strategies for engaging nurses. Journal of Nursing Administration (2014), 44(3), 142-151.

40. Reimer, N., & Herbener, L.; Round and round we go: Rounding strategies to impact exemplary professional practice. Clinical Journal of Oncology Nursing (2014), 18(6), 654-660.

41. Meade, C. M., Kennedy, J., & Kaplan, J.; The effects of emergency department staff rounding on patient safety and satisfaction. Journal of Emergency Medicine (2010), 38(5), 666-674.

42. Nash, M., Pestrue, J., Geier, P., Sharp, K., Helder, A., & McAlearney, A. S. Leveraging information technology to drive improvement in patient satisfaction. Journal of Healthcare Quality (2010), 32(5), 30-40.

43. Sharieff GQ, Burnell L, Cantonis M, Norton V, Tovar J, Roberts K, VanWyk C, Saucier J, Russe J.; Improving emergency department time to provider, left-without-treatment rates, and average length of stay. J Emerg Med. 2013 Sep; 45(3):426-32.

44. Liselotte N. Dyrbye, Tait D. Shanafelt; Physician Burnout A Potential Threat to Successful Health Care Reform. JAMA, May 18, 2011—Vol 305, No. 19.

45. Michael D Brundage, Claire F Snyder; Patient-reported outcomes in clinical practice: using standards to break down barriers. Clin. Invest. (2012) 2(4), 343–346.

46. Ethan Basch; Patient-Reported Outcomes — Harnessing Patients' Voices to Improve Clinical Care. The New England Journal of Medicine, January 12, 2017, 376;2.

47. Lisa S. Rotenstein, Robert S. Huckman, & Neil W. Wagle; Making Patients and Doctors Happier — The Potential of Patient-Reported Outcomes. The New England Journal of Medicine, October 2017, 377;14.

48. Pakhomov SV, Jacobsen SJ, Chute CG, Roger VL. Agreement between patient-reported symptoms and their documentation in the medical record. Am J Manag Care. 2008; 14: 530-9.

49. Wu AW, Kharrazi H, Boulware LE, Snyder CF. Measure once, cut twice — adding Symptom management is a cornerstone of clinical care, patient-reported outcome measures to the electronic health record for comparative effectiveness research. J Clin Epidemiol 2013;66: Suppl: S12-S20.

50. Snyder CF, Aaronson NK, Choucair AK, et al. Implementing patient-reported outcomes assessment in clinical practice: a review of the options and considerations. Qual Life Res 2012; 21: 1305-14.

51. Kotronoulas G, Kearney N, Maguire R, et al. What is the value of the routine use of patient-reported outcome measures toward improvement of patient outcomes, processes of care, and health service outcomes in cancer care? A systematic review of controlled trials. J Clin Oncol 2014; 32: 1480-501.

52. Basch E, Deal AM, Kris MG, et al. Symptom monitoring with patient-reported outcomes during routine cancer treatment: a randomized controlled trial. J Clin Oncol 2016; 34: 557-65.

53. Alexandra Soroceanu, Alexander Ching, William Abdu, Kevin McGuire; Relationship between Preoperative Expectations, and Postoperative Satisfaction and Functional Outcomes in Lumbar and Cervical Spine Patients: A Multicenter Study. The spine journal, October 2011Volume 11, Issue 10, Supplement, Page S75.

54. Andreas Kiilerich Andresen, et al; Patient-reported outcomes and patient-reported satisfaction after surgical treatment for cervical radiculopathy. Global Spine Journal, P 1-6, 2018.

55. Findik, U. Y., Unsar, S. & Sut, N.; Patient satisfaction with nursing care and its relationship with patient characteristics. Nursing and Health Sciences (2010). 12(2), 162-169.

56. Tonio Schoenfelder, Jörg Klewer, Joachim Kugler; Determinants of Patient Satisfaction: A Study among 39 Hospitals in an In-Patient Setting in Germany. International Journal for Quality in Health Care 2011; Volume 23, Number 5: pp. 503–509.

57. Witiw CD, Mansouri A, Mathieu F, Nassiri F, Badhiwala JH, et al. Exploring the expectation-actuality discrepancy: a systematic review of the impact of preoperative expectations on satisfaction and patient reported outcomes in spinal surgery. (2016) Neurosurg Rev, pp: 1-12.

58. Akhila Sure, Jared C Tishelman, John Moon, Peter Zhou and Subaraman Ramchandran; Patient reported satisfaction and its impact on outcomes in spinal surgery: A mini review. Annals of Clinical and Laboratory Research. 2016 Vol.4 No.3:115.

59. Sigmundsson FG, Jönsson B, Strömqvist B; Determinants of patient satisfaction after surgery for central spinal stenosis without concomitant spondylolisthesis: a register study of 5100 patients. Eur Spine J, (2016). Vol. (26), pp: 473-480.

60. Mannion AF, Junge A, Elfering A, Dvorak J, Porchet F, et al. Great expectations: really the novel predictor of outcome after spinal surgery? (2009) Spine (Phila Pa 1976) 34: 1590-1599.

61. Mancuso CA, Duculan R, Cammisa FP; Fulfillment of patients' expectations of lumbar and cervical spine surgery. Spine J. 2016 Oct;16(10):1167-1174.

62. Kenneth Sands and Lauge Sokol-Hessner; Patient-Centered Care. Principles and Practice of Hospital Medicine, Second Edition. 2017 by McGraw-Hill Education. P 104-109.

63. VanLare JM, Conway PH: Value-based purchasing—national programs to move from volume to value. N Engl J Med. 367:292–295, 2012.

64. Petrullo KA, Lamar S, Nwankwo-Otti O, Alexander-Mills K, Viola D: The Patient Satisfaction Survey: What does it mean to your bottom line? J Hosp Adm 2:1–8, 2013.

65. Jay M. Levin, Robert D. Winkelman, Joseph E. Tanenbaum, Edward C. Benzel, Thomas E. Mroz, and Michael P. Steinmetz; Key drivers of patient satisfaction in lumbar spine surgery. J Neurosurg Spine 28:586–592, 2018.

66. Machado GC, Ferreira PH, Harris IA, Pinheiro MB, Koes BW, van Tulder M, et al: Effectiveness of surgery for lumbar spinal stenosis: a systematic review and meta-analysis. PLoS One 10:e0122800, 2015.

67. Clifford Bleustein, et al; Wait Times, Patient Satisfaction Scores, and the Perception of Care. Am J Manag Care. 2014; 20(5):393-400.

68. Shilpa Darivemula; John Huppertz, and Elena Rosenbaum; Decreasing Wait Times in a Family Medicine Clinic -A Creative Approach. Family Doctor. A Journal of the New York State Academy of Family Physicians, Summer 2016. Volume five. Number one.

69. Fabian Camacho, et al; The Relationship between Patient's Perceived Waiting Time and Office-Based Practice Satisfaction. NC Med J November/December 2006, Volume 67, Number 6.

70. Nemschoff Insight, Winning Strategies for Waiting Rooms, 2015, report available from http://www.nemschoff.com/uploads/case-study files/Nemschoff_Insight_Winning_Strategies_for_Waiting_Rooms_2015_01_13.pdf.

71. Shah, Shital; Patel, Anay; Rumoro, Dino P.; Hohmann, Samuel; and Fullam, Francis (2015) "Managing patient expectations at emergency department triage. Patient Experience Journal, Volume 2, Issue 2 - Fall 2015.

72. Diane Glowacki; Effective pain management and improvements in patients' outcomes and satisfaction. CriticalCareNurse Vol 35, No. 3, JUNE 2015. P 33-41.

73. Breivik H. Postoperative pain management: why is it difficult to show that it improves outcomes? Eur J Anaesthesiol. 1998;15(6):748-751].

74. Twersky R, Fishman D, Homel P. What happens after discharge? Return hospital visits after ambulatory surgery. Anesth Analg. 1997;84(2):319-324.

75. Carr DB, Goudas LC. Acute pain. Lancet. 1999; 353(9169):2051-2058.

76. Wells N, Pasero C, McCaffery M. Improving the quality of care through pain assessment and management. In: Hughes RG, ed. Patient Safety and Quality: An Evidence-Based Handbook for Nurses. Rockville, MD: US Agency for Healthcare Research and Quality; 2008:469-497.

77. Gan TJ, Habib AS, Miller TE, White W, Apfelbaum JL.; Incidence, patient satisfaction, and perceptions of post-surgical pain: results from a US national survey. Curr Med Res Opin. 2014 Jan;30(1):149-60.

78. Pathmawathi S, Beng TS, Li LM, Rosli R, Sharwend S, Kavitha RR, Christopher BC.; Satisfaction with and perception of pain management among palliative patients with breakthrough pain: A qualitative study. Pain Manag Nurs. 2015 Aug;16(4):552-60.

79. Apfelbaum JL, Chen C, Mehta SS, Gan TJ: Postoperative pain experience: results from a national survey suggest postoperative pain continues to be undermanaged. Anesth Analg 97:534–540, 2003.

80. Miller J, Dunion A, Dunn N, Fitzmaurice C, Gamboa M, Myers S, Novak P, Poole J, Rice K, Riley C, Sandberg R, Taylor D, Gilmore L.; Effect of a brief massage on pain, anxiety, and satisfaction with pain management in postoperative orthopaedic patients. Orthop Nurs. 2015 Jul-Aug; 34(4):227-34.

81. Botelho RJ, Lue BH, Fiscella K.; Family involvement in routine health care: a survey of patients' behaviors and preferences. J Fam Pract. 1996 Jun; 42(6):572-6.

82. Jennifer L. Wolff, Cynthia M. Boyd, Laura N. Gitlin, Martha L. Bruce, and Debra L. Roter; Going it together; Persistence of older adults' accompaniment to physician visits by a family companion. J Am Geriatr Soc. 2012 January ; 60(1): 106–112.

83. Locatelli SM, Hill JN, Bokhour BG, Krejci L, Fix GM, Nora Mueller, Solomon JL, Van Deusen Lukas C, LaVela SL.; Provider perspectives on and experiences with engagement of patients and families in implementing patient-centered care. Healthc (Amst). 2015 Dec;3(4):209-14.

84. Jennifer L. Wolff, Marla L. Clayman, Peter Rabins MD, Mary Ann Cook, and Debra L. Roter; An exploration of patient and family engagement in routine primary care visits. Health Expectations, 18, pp.188–198. 2012 John Wiley & Sons Ltd.

85. Mary T Shannon ; Please hear what I'm not saying: The art of listening in the clinical encounter. The Permanente Journal/ Spring 2011/ Volume 15 No. 2. PP e114-e117.

86. Cox ME, Yancy WS Jr, Coffman CJ, et al. Effects of counseling techniques on patients' weight related attitudes and behaviors in a primary care clinic. Patient Educ Couns. Feb 11.2011 Epub ahead of print.

87. Fogarty LA, Curbow BA, Wingard JR, McDonnell K, Somerfield MR. Can 40 seconds of compassion reduce patient anxiety? J Clin Oncol. 1999; 17:371–9.

88. Kathryn I. Pollak, et al; Physician empathy and listening: associations with patient satisfaction and autonomy. J Am Board Fam Med. 2011 Nov; 24(6): 665–672.

89. Paul M Arnold, et al; Factors affecting hospital length of stay following anterior cervical discectomy and fusion. Evidence Based Spine Care Journal. Volume2/Issue3—2011. P 11-18.

90. http://hcahpsonline.org

91. HCAHPS best practices in high performing critical access hospitals. May 2017. Stratis Health Rural Quality Improvement Technical Assistance | www.stratishealth.org.

92. Karen Cook; HCAHPS update and impacting the patient perception of care. Webinar presented on January 28, 2009. Hackensack University Medical Center. www.studergroup.com.

93. Toma G, Triner W, McNutt L. Patient satisfaction as a function of emergency department previsit expectations. Annals of Emergency Medicine 2009;54(3):360-367.

94. Altringer B. The emotional experience of patient care: a case for innovation in health care design. J Health Serv Res Policy 2010; 15(3):174-177.

95. Lown BA, Manning CF. The Schwartz Center Rounds: Evaluation of an interdisciplinary approach to enhancing patient-centered communication, teamwork, and provider support. Academic Medicine 2010; 85(6):1073-1081.

96. Whitney McKnight; Nurse Leadership Development Tied Directly to Improved Patient and Staff Experience Ratings. Press Ganey Publication | March 2017.

97. Sukhminder Jit Singh Bajwa and Rudrashish Haldar; Pain management following spinal surgeries; An appraisal of available options. J Craniovertebr Junction Spine. 2015 Jul-Sep; 6(3): 105–110.

98. Jad Bou Monsef, Fernando Techy; Patient selection for spine surgery. Benzel's spine surgery, techniques, complication avoidance, and management. Fourth edition. 2017 by Elsevier. P 219-220.

99. Daniel J. Ellis, et al; The Relationship between Preoperative Expectations and the Short-Term Postoperative Satisfaction and Functional Outcome in Lumbar Spine Surgery: A Systematic Review. Global Spine J 2015; 5:436–452.

100. Yee A, Adjei N, Do J, Ford M, Finkelstein J.; Do patient expectations of spinal surgery relate to functional outcome? Clin Orthop Relat Res 2008; 466(5):1154–1161.

101. Saniya S. Godil, et al; Determining the quality and effectiveness of surgical spine care: patient satisfaction is not a valid proxy. Spine J. 2013 Sep; 13(9):1006-12.

102. Tomoaki Toyone, et al; Patients' expectations and satisfaction in lumbar spine surgery. Spine. 30(23):2689-2694, DEC 2005.

103. Chotai S, Sivaganesan A, Parker SL, McGirt MJ, Devin CJ.; Patient-specific factors associated with dissatisfaction after elective surgery for degenerative spine diseases. Neurosurgery. 2015 Aug;77(2):157-63.

104. Alexandra Soroceanu; Alexander Ching; William Abdu; Kevin McGuire; Relationship between preoperative expectations, satisfaction, and functional outcomes in patients undergoing lumbar and cervical spine surgery: a multicenter study. Spine. 37(2):E103–E108, JAN 2012.

105. Basem I. Awad, Thomas E. Mroz, Michael P. Steinmetz; Minimal access and percutaneous lumbar discectomy. Benzel's spine surgery, techniques, complication avoidance, and management. Fourth edition. 2017 by Elsevier. P 774-782.

106. Roberto Casal-Moro, et al; Long-term outcome after Microendoscopic diskectomy for lumbar disk herniation: A prospective clinical study with a 5-year follow-up. Neurosurgery 68:1568–1575, 2011.

107. Raul A. Vasquez, et al; The profile of a smoker and its impact on outcomes after cervical spine surgery. Neurosurgery, Volume 63, Issue CN_suppl_1, 1 August 2016, Pages 96–101.

108. Freyr Gauti Sigmundsson, Bo Jönsson and Björn Strömqvist; Determinants of patient satisfaction after surgery for central spinal stenosis without concomitant spondylolisthesis: a register study of 5100 patients. European Spine Journal. February 2017, Volume 26, Issue 2, pp 473–480.

109. Sandén B, Försth P, Michaëlsson K (2011) Smokers show less improvement than nonsmokers two years after surgery for lumbar spinal stenosis: a study of 4555 patients from the Swedish spine register. Spine 36:1059–1064.

110. Godil SS, Parker SL, Zuckerman SL, Mendenhall SK, Devin CJ, Asher A et al; Determining the quality and effectiveness of surgical spine care: patient satisfaction is not a valid proxy (2013). Spine J 13(9):1006–1012.

111. Laura Chapin; Kelly Ward, Timothy Ryken; Preoperative depression, smoking, and employment status are significant factors in patient satisfaction after lumbar spine surgery. Clinical Spine Surgery. 30(6):E725–E732, JUL 2017.

112. Charles H. Crawford III, et al; Impact of preoperative diagnosis on patient satisfaction following lumbar spine surgery. Journal of Neurosurgery: Spine. Jun 2017 / Vol. 26 / No. 6 / Pages 709-715.

113. Alrawi MF, Khalil NM, Mitchell P, Hughes SP. The value of neurophysiological and imaging studies in predicting outcome in the surgical treatment of cervical radiculopathy. Eur Spine J. Apr 2007;16(4):495-500.

114. Sapan D. Gandhi; Kristen E. Radcliff; Obesity in lumbar spine surgery. Current Orthopaedic Practice. 27(2):135–139, MAR 2016.

115. Knutsson B, Michaëlsson K, Sandén B: Obesity is associated with inferior results after surgery for lumbar spinal stenosis: a study of 2633 patients from the Swedish spine register. Spine (Phila Pa 1976) 38:435–441, 2013.

116. McGuire KJ, et al: The effect of high obesity on outcomes of treatment for lumbar spinal conditions: subgroup analysis of the spine patient outcomes research trial. Spine (Phila Pa 1976) 39:1975–1980, 2014.

117. Cinzia Gaudelli, Ken Thomas; Obesity and early reoperation rate after elective lumbar spine surgery: a population based study. Evidence-Based Spine-Care Journal. Volume 3/Issue 2. 2012. P 11-16.

118. Aalto TJ, et al: Preoperative predictors for postoperative clinical outcome in lumbar spinal stenosis: systematic review. Spine (Phila Pa 1976) 31:E648–E663, 2006.

119. Andrew K. Chan, et al; Women fare best following surgery for degenerative lumbar spondylolisthesis: a comparison of the most and least satisfied patients utilizing data from the Quality Outcomes Database. Neurosurg Focus 44 (1):E3, 2018.

120. Elsamadicy AA, et al: Impact of gender disparities on short-term and long-term patient reported outcomes and satisfaction measures after elective lumbar spine surgery: a single institutional study of 384 patients. World Neurosurg 107:952–958, 2017.

121. Shabat S, et al: Gender differences as an influence on patients' satisfaction rates in spinal surgery of elderly patients. Eur Spine J 14:1027–1032. 2005.

122. Levin JM, Winkelman RD, Smith GA, Tanenbaum JE, Benzel EC, Mroz TE, et al: Impact of preoperative depression on hospital consumer assessment of healthcare providers and systems survey results in a lumbar fusion population. Spine (Phila Pa 1976) 42:675–681, 2017.

123. Robert K. Merrill; Lukas P. Zebala; Colleen Peters; Sheeraz A. Qureshi; Steven J. McAnany; Impact of depression on patient-reported outcome measures after lumbar spine decompression. SPINE. 43(6):434–439, MAR 2018.

124. Mannion AF, Fekete TF, Porchet F, Haschtmann D, Jeszenszky D, Kleinstück FS: The influence of comorbidity on the risks and benefits of spine surgery for degenerative lumbar disorders. Eur Spine J 23 (Suppl 1):S66–S71, 2014.

125. Harminder Singh, George M. Ghobrial, Shannon W. Hann, James S. Harrop; Fundamentals of spine surgery. Benzel's spine surgery, techniques, complication avoidance, and management. Fourth edition. 2017 by Elsevier. P 206.

126. Slosar PJ, et al; Patient satisfaction after circumferential lumbar fusion. Spine (Phila Pa 1976). 2000 Mar 15; 25(6):722-6.

127. Hasan Ghandehari, et al; Evaluation of patient outcome and satisfaction after surgical treatment of adolescent idiopathic scoliosis using scoliosis research society-30. Arch Bone Jt Surg. 2015 Apr; 3(2): 109–113.

128. Carreon LY, et al; Patient satisfaction after surgical correction of adolescent idiopathic scoliosis. Spine (Phila Pa 1976). 2011 May 20;36(12):965-8.

129. E. Ameri, et al; Patient satisfaction after scoliosis surgery. Medical Journal of the Islamic Republic of Iran.Vol. 21, No. 4, February 2008. pp. 177-184.

130. Jin-Young Lee, Seong-Hwan Moon, Bo-Kyung Suh, Myung Ho Yang, and Moon Soo Park; Outcome and complications in surgical treatment of lumbar stenosis or spondylolisthesis in geriatric patients. Yonsei Med J 2015 Sep; 56(5):1199-1205.

131. Glassman SD, Polly DW, Bono CM, Burkus K, Dimar JR. Outcome of lumbar arthrodesis in patients sixty-five years of age or older. J Bone Joint Surg Am 2009; 91: 783-90.

132. Glassman SD, Carreon LY, Dimar JR, Campbell MJ, Puno RM, Johnson JR. Clinical outcomes in older patients after posterolateral lumbar fusion. Spine J 2007; 7: 547-51.

133. Noboru Hosono, Kazuo Yonenobu; Cervical Laminoplasty. Benzel's spine surgery techniques, complication avoidance, and management. Fourth edition. 2017 by Elsevier. P 699-705.

134. Yasuhiro Takeshima, et al; Surgical outcome of laminoplasty for cervical spondylotic myelopathy in an elderly population – potentiality for effective early surgical intervention: A meta-analysis. Neurol Med Chir (Tokyo) 57,366–373, 2017.

135. Nan Su, et al; Long-term outcomes and prognostic analysis of modified open-door laminoplasty with lateral mass screw fusion in treatment of cervical spondylotic myelopathy. Therapeutics and Clinical Risk Management 2016:12 1329–1337.

136. Fukui M, Chiba K, Kawakami M, et al. JOA Back Pain Evaluation Questionnaire (JOABPEQ)/JOA Cervical Myelopathy Evaluation Questionnaire (JOACMEQ): the report on the development of revised versions. J Orthop Sci. 2009;14: 348-365.

137. Handa Y, Kubota T, Ishii H, et al. Evaluation of prognostic factors and clinical outcome in elderly patients in whom expansive laminoplasty is performed for cervical myelopathy due to multisegmental spondylotic canal stenosis: a retrospective comparison with younger patients. J Neurosurg. 2002; 96(suppl 2): 173-179.

138. Okuda S, Oda T, Miyauchi A, et al. Surgical outcomes of posterior lumbar interbody fusion in elderly patients: surgical technique. J Bone Joint Surg Am. 2007; 89(suppl 2):310-320.

139. Atsushi Kimura, Teruaki Endo, Hirokazu Inoue, Atsushi Seichi. Preoperative predictors of patient satisfaction with outcome after cervical laminoplasty. Global Spine J 2014; 4:77–82.

140. Park Y and Ha JW. Comparison of one-level posterior lumbar interbody fusion performed with a minimally invasive approach or a traditional open approach. Spine. 2007; 32:537-543.

141. Eleftherios Archavlis, Mario Carvi y Nievas; Comparison of minimally invasive fusion and instrumentation versus open surgery for severe stenotic spondylolisthesis with high-grade facet joint osteoarthritis. Eur Spine J. 2013 Aug; 22(8): 1731–1740.

142. Praveen V. Mummaneni, et al; Minimally invasive versus open fusion for Grade I degenerative lumbar spondylolisthesis: analysis of the Quality Outcomes Database. Neurosurg Focus 43 (2):E11, 2017.

143. Lu VM, Kerezoudis P, Gilder HE, McCutcheon BA, Phan K, Bydon M: Minimally invasive surgery versus open surgery spinal fusion for spondylolisthesis: a systematic review and meta-analysis. Spine (Phila Pa 1976) 42:E177–E185, 2017.

144. Parker SL, Mendenhall SK, Shau DN, Zuckerman SL, Godil SS, Cheng JS, et al: Minimally invasive versus open transforaminal lumbar interbody fusion for degenerative spondylolisthesis: comparative effectiveness and cost-utility analysis. World Neurosurg 82:230–238, 2014.

145. Giuseppe MV Barbagallo, Emily Yoder, Joseph R Dettori, Vincenzo Albanese; Percutaneous minimally invasive versus open spine surgery in the treatment of fractures of the thoracolumbar junction: a comparative effectiveness review. Evidence-Based Spine-Care Journal. Volume 3/Issue 3 -2012. P 43-49.

146. Ron Riesenburger, Paul Klimo Jr., Mina G. Safain, Edward C. Benzel; Motion-Sparing, Nonimplant Surgery: Cervical Spine and Lumbar Spine. Benzel's spine surgery, techniques, complication avoidance, and management. Fourth edition. 2017 by Elsevier. P 1575-1580.

147. Todd B. Francis, Edward C. Benzel; Biomechanics of motion preservation techniques. Benzel's spine surgery, techniques, complication avoidance, and management. Fourth edition. 2017 by Elsevier. P 1581-1586.e1.

148. Frank M. Phillips, et al; Long-term Outcomes of the US FDA IDE prospective, randomized controlled clinical trial comparing PCM cervical disc arthroplasty with anterior cervical discectomy and fusion. SPINE Volume 40, Number 10, pp 674 – 683. 2015.

149. Phillips FM, Lee JY, Geisler FH, et al. A prospective, randomized, controlled clinical investigation comparing PCM cervical disc arthroplasty with anterior cervical discectomy and fusion. 2-year results from the US FDA IDE clinical trial. Spine 2013; 38: E907 – 18.

150. Zigler JE, Delamarter R, Murrey D, et al. ProDisc-C and anterior cervical discectomy and fusion as surgical treatment for single-level cervical symptomatic degenerative disc disease: five-year results of a Food and Drug Administration study. Spine 2013; 38: 203 – 9.

151. Murrey D, Janssen M, Delamarter R, et al. Results of the prospective, randomized, controlled multicenter Food and Drug Administration investigational device exemption study of the ProDisc-C total disc replacement versus anterior discectomy and fusion for the treatment of 1-level symptomatic cervical disc disease. Spine J. Apr 2009; 9(4):275-286.

152. NASS Clinical Guidelines – Diagnosis and treatment of cervical radiculopathy from degenerative disorders. 2010 North American Spine Society. P-66.

153. Park DK, et al. Does multilevel lumbar stenosis lead to poorer outcomes? A subanalysis of the Spine Patient Outcomes Research Trial (SPORT) lumbar stenosis study. Spine (Phila Pa 1976). 2010; 35 (4):439-46.

154. Amundsen T, Weber H, Nordal HJ, Magnaes B, Abdelnoor M, Lilleås F.; Lumbar spinal stenosis: conservative or surgical management?: A prospective 10-year study. Spine (Phila Pa 1976) 2000; 25(11):1424-35; discussion 1435-6.

155. North American Spine Society. Clinical guidelines for multidisciplinary spine care, diagnosis and treatment of degenerative lumbar spinal stenosis. 2011. P 9.

156. Zeev Arinzon, Abraham Adunsky, Zeev Fidelman, and Reuven Gepstein; Outcomes of decompression surgery for lumbar spinal stenosis in elderly diabetic patients. Eur Spine J. 2004; 13(1): 32-7.

157. North American Spine Society. Clinical guidelines for multidisciplinary spine care. Diagnosis and treatment of degenerative lumbar spinal stenosis. 2011. P 56-63.

158. Arinzon ZH, et al. Surgical management of spinal stenosis: a comparison of immediate and long term outcome in two geriatric patient populations. Arch Gerontol Geriatr. 2003; 36(3): 273-9.

Appendix I

Data show presentation on the
subject of patient satisfaction
(Delivered on the 3rd International
Conference on Spine and Spinal Disorders,
June 11-13, 2018 London, UK)

PATIENT SATISFACTION IN SPINE PRACTICE

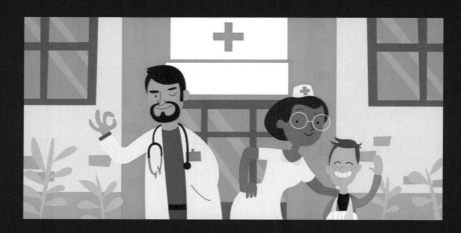

T A Hamdan, FRCS, FRCP, FACS, FICS,
American Board (Nevada)
Professor Orthopaedic Surgery
Basrah-Iraq.

In Cambridge
English dictionary,
satisfaction is

- A pleasant feeling that you get when you receive something you wanted or when you have done something you wanted to do.

Or

- A situation in which your complaint or problem is dealt with in a way you considered acceptable.

- Richard L. and sholasky 2018 define patient satisfaction

As the degree to which a patient feels that they have received high quality health care

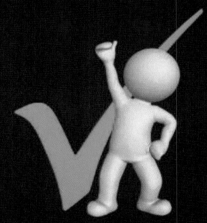

- Pascoe GC. 1983 describe satisfaction;

Satisfaction can be described as patient reaction to several service experience

Vital points

- Many writers start differentiating between treatment offered and satisfaction achieved
- Patient satisfaction is a top priority
- Perfect treatment not always leads to satisfaction
- At some stations, satisfaction may be broken

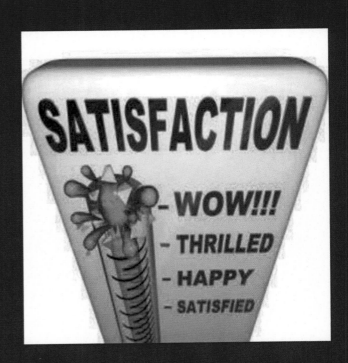

Vital points

- The treating physician is always the target
- The art of communication and patient handling is not that easy
- In general it is either medical or non medical

Satisfaction percentage was very variable, so far no fixed number

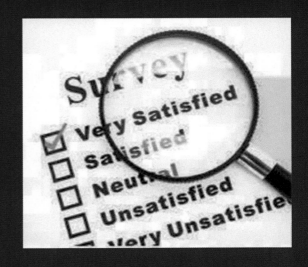

Reported

- 66% of patients with primary disc herniation and 67% with spondylolisthesis reported their expectation were met,
- lower proportion with stenosis and adjacent segment disease.

Patient expectation and satisfaction (Toyone Tomoaki et al. 2005)

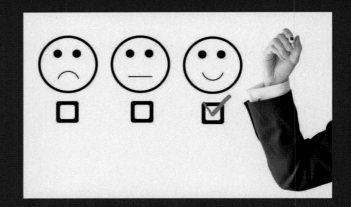

Conclusion

- Even if the clinical expectation were met, some patients were still dissatisfied
- Patients with spinal stenosis seem to have more unrealistic expectations than patients with disc prolapse

The trouble makers
(odd patients)

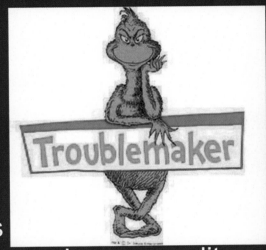

- Terminally ill patients
- Uninsured and poor patients
- Mentally ill, abnormal psyche, rushy personality
- Bed ridden patients
- Poor education standards
- VIP, top officials or VVIP
- Patients with associated other chronic illness (renal, cardiac, collagen disease,…)

The relation between preoperative expectation and satisfaction (soroceanu et al. 2013)

- Expectation dramatically affect spine patient satisfaction
- Greater fulfilment of expectation leads to higher postoperative satisfaction

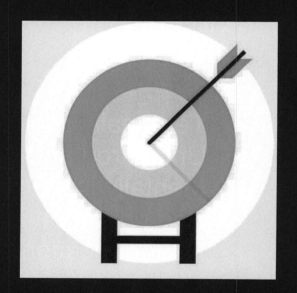

The relation between preoperative expectation and satisfaction (Soroceanu et al. 2013)

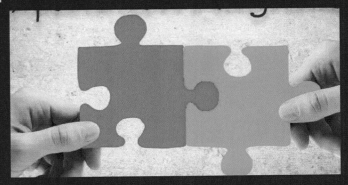

- Higher preoperative expectations leads to decreased postsurgical satisfaction but was associated with improved functional outcome
- Preoperative expectation should be considered to obtain an informed choice on the basis of patients preference.

The impact of preoperative diagnosis on patient satisfaction following lumbar spine surgery (Crawford Ch. Et al, 2017)

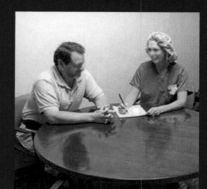

- A greater proportion of patients with primary disc prolapse or spondylolisthesis reported that surgery met expectation (66% and 67%)
- While recurrent herniation and stenosis (59%, 60%)
- A smaller proportion of patients who underwent surgery for adjacent segment degeneration or mechanical disc collapse had expectation met (48% and 41%)

Surgeon related and
facilities related

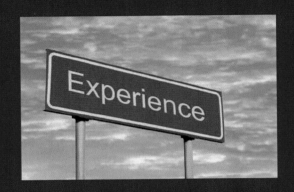

- The competence and past experience in this particular field
- The humanistic handling
- The ability to clarify every thing in gentle way (the art of communication)
- Up to date surgeon
- Sharing opinions with colleagues
- The availability of the specified facilities for the specified pathology.

Patient related factors (Richard L
schlocky 2018)

- Satisfaction is highly
  dependent on patient
  expectation
- This can be achieved if the
  patient and surgeon are
  provided with factual
  probabilities of achieving
  better or worse outcome
- Individual risk factors should
  be identified prior to surgery

Patient related factors (Richard L schlocky 2018)

- Devin: insist that spine care provider should consider that patients who fail to achieve clinically significant outcome, those with Medicaid or uninsured and those presenting with worse pain and disability were less likely to satisfied.

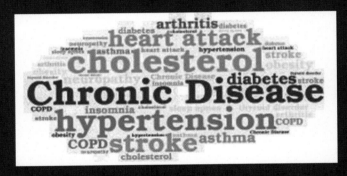

Godil SS., parker SL., Zukerman SL. (2013) conclude:

- Patient satisfaction is not a valid proxy in determining the quality and effectiveness of surgical spine care

While Mannion et al. (2009)

- Suggest that great expectation that novel predictor of outcome after spinal surgery

M. Bydon et al. (2016)

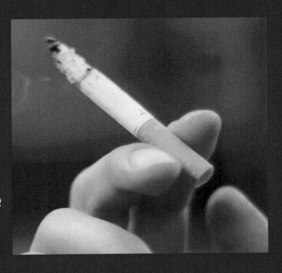

- Smoking has been associated with worse self reported outcome
- Smoking is a significant risk factor for complications
- Tobacco lead to delay tissue healing
- So smoking is a negative predictor of outcome

Can we predict satisfaction in the preoperative period?

The answer almost yes depending on the following parameters:

- The personality
- Psychologic background
- Site of lesion/ multiple or single
- The nature of pathology
- The pattern of surgery
- Previous spine surgery
- The behavior of previous colleagues
- Site pain
- The degree of disability
- The patient expectation

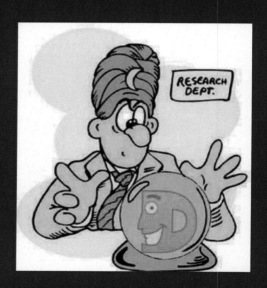

Probably knowing if patient will be willing to undergo the same procedure is an indicator of satisfaction

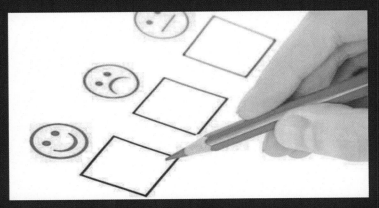

According to Laura Dedra et al. 2017

The result is following:
1. Disc herniation: 88%
2. Spondylolisthesis: 86%
3. Stenosis: 82%
4. Recurrent disc: 79%
5. Adjacent segment disease: 75%
6. Mechanical collapse: 73%

Determinants of patients
satisfaction after surgery for central
canal stenosis without
spondylolisthesis (a study of 5100
patients)

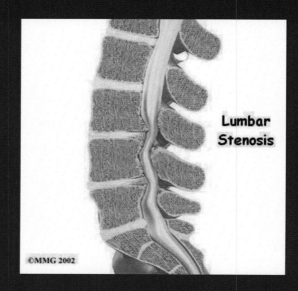

- Numerous factors have predictive value for satisfaction of outcome after surgery for central canal stenosis
- Factors decreasing likelihood for satisfaction include previous surgery, smoking, unemployment, back pain exceeding one year, back pain predominance, preoperative self estimated walking distance
- (European spine journal 2016)

Patient satisfaction after circumferential lumbar fusion (Slosarj et al. 2000)

They conclude that:
- Circumferential lumbar fusion is a useful procedure with very high fusion rate
- Overall 62% of patients are satisfied with the result
- Patients who are working before surgery and patients who are not injured workers also tended to progress well

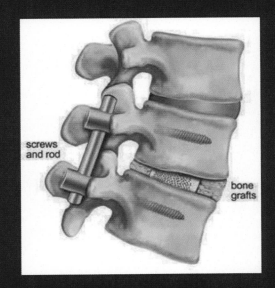

Patient satisfaction after circumferential lumbar fusion (Slosarj et al. 2000)

- 11% choose the statement: surgery met my expectation
- 51% surgery improve my condition
- 26% surgery helped
- 19% I am the same or worse compared with before surgery

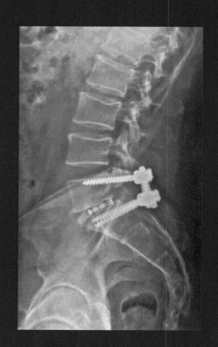

In chines cohort study by (Wang et al. 2015)

- The factors predicting patients satisfaction were
- More than 70% patients expressed satisfaction with discectomy
- Two factors could predict patient dissatisfaction and be assessed before surgery: obesity and preoperative depression
- Symptoms recurrence and postoperative depression are also associated with diminished patient satisfaction.

Satisfaction after scoliosis surgery (E. Ameri 2008)

- Those with severe curve only 50% were satisfied
- After combined anterior and posterior fusion, showed greater dissatisfaction if compared with posterior fusion alone

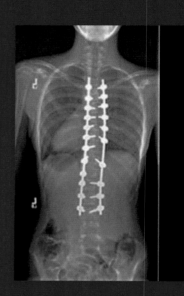

Satisfaction after scoliosis surgery (E. Ameri 2008)

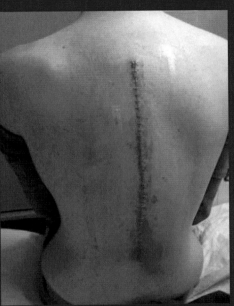

- Neutral or dissatisfaction were more likely to have with king II or king IV curve
- Preoperative physical characteristic psychological difficulties and unrealistic expectation regarding postoperative cosmoses are associated with patient neutralizing or dissatisfaction

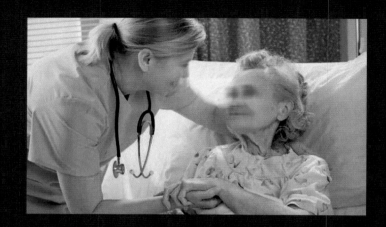

In one study

- 66% of patients with primary disc herniation and 67% with spondylolisthesis reported their expectation were met lower proportion with stenosis and adjacent segment disease

Take home messages

- Proper prolong preoperative evaluation of the patient status is mandatory
- The pathology had a lot to do with patient satisfaction
- Several parameters have also impact on satisfaction even if not related to the pathology like depression, employment, insurance and so on
- What patients expect from spine surgery is important as it relates to patient satisfaction

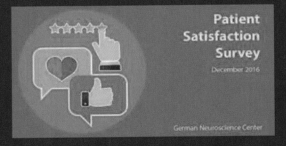

Take home messages

- Even if the clinical expectations were met some patients will be dissatisfied
- Patients with spinal stenosis seems to have more unrealistic expectation, same with deformity
- The surgeon experience and capability and theatre facilities plays important rule in achieving satisfaction
- Chose the right patient for spinal surgery

Some points that may help in satisfaction or dissatisfaction

- Handling of previous colleagues
- Previous experience with hospitals
- The background feeling of health service
- His pain response
- The length of the waiting list
- The nature of the pathology
- Previous response to treatment

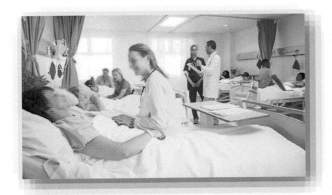

Probably useful to ask the following questions to the patient prior to treatment

- What do you think about our services?
- What do you expect me to do for you?
- Why you have chosen me and this hospital?

The cornerstone is the treating physician

- He is everything for the good and bad outcome
- The first meeting, either salt in the wound or long life friendship
- The response to patient suffering
- His reputation

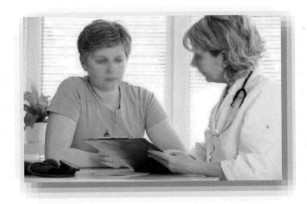

- How impressive was the physician
- Can the physician implants confidence and respect in the patient's mind
- The physician scientific background
- Previous colleagues mishandling and mistakes

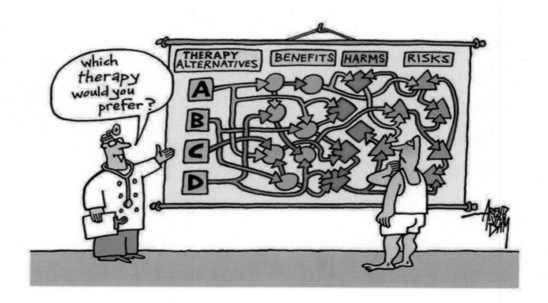

Satisfaction factors

(Poor, Good, Very Good, Excellent)

- Reception response
- Ward environment
- Food offered
- Laboratory results
- The physician attitude
- Time given for answering questions
- Facilities available in general
- Nursing and porters staff

Thank you

Printed in the United States
By Bookmasters